Expanding Nursing and Health Care Practice

Series Editor: Lynne Wigens

Interprofessional Working

An essential guide for health- and social-care professionals

Jane Day

Nelson Thornes

Kluwer business

Published in 2006 by:
Nelson Thornes Ltd
Delta Place
27 Bath Road
CHELTENHAM
GL53 7TH
United Kingdom

08 09 10 / 10 9 8 7 6 5 4 3 2

A catalogue record for this book is available from the British Library

ISBN 978-0-7487-9768-4

Cover photograph by Stockbyte RF (NT)
Illustrations by Florence Production Ltd, Stoodleigh, Devon
Page make-up by Florence Production Ltd, Stoodleigh, Devon

Printed and bound by GraphyCems, Spain

Contents

Acknowledgements		iv
Preface		v
Chapter 1	Introduction – The key concepts of interprofessional working	1
Chapter 2	The context of interprofessional working	13
Chapter 3	Teams, teamwork and team dynamics	33
Chapter 4	Leadership and expertise	55
Chapter 5	Communicating with each other	81
Chapter 6	Interprofessional learning within a practice environment	106
Chapter 7	Barriers to effective interprofessional working	131
Appendix	Rapid recap answers	155
Index		161

Acknowledgements

I would like to take this opportunity to thank my friends and colleagues who helped and supported me while I wrote this book. I would particularly like to thank colleagues in both the Faculty of Health, Suffolk College and health- and social-care professionals from the practice setting who have provided practice scenarios, case studies and their thoughts on aspects of interprofessional working for inclusion in this book.

Preface

Over recent years the need for health- and social-care professionals to work in different ways has become ever more evident as the context within which health and social care is delivered has changed. The momentum towards interprofessional working has increased significantly since the late 1990s, when the White Paper, *The New NHS, Modern – Dependable* (Secretary of State for Health, 1997) was published. This White Paper began a programme of modernisation on a scale that had not been seen in the NHS since it was set up in 1948. There was now a clear commitment by the government to make the patient the focus of modern health- and social-care services. The achievement of this will require radical reform of services and reform of the workforce.

Changes affecting the workforce have already taken place, for example the development of new and specialised roles and the introduction of a new pay system. These changes will continue to occur as the workforce develops and evolves. Traditional professional boundaries are being challenged, as health- and social-care professionals cross the boundaries to deliver patient-focused care using a team approach. To support these new ways of working, there have been radical changes to the education and training of health- and social-care professionals at both pre- and post-qualifying levels. The emphasis is on the interprofessional learning, with different professionals learning with, from and about each other in order to improve collaboration and thus enhance the quality of care provided. Significant organisational changes have also taken place to enable different agencies, notably, but not exclusively, the health services and social services, to work more effectively together.

Health- and social-care delivery is constantly in the spotlight and hardly a day goes by without the media making reference to a change that is proposed or has taken place. Sadly, all too often the media are reporting the tragic death of a vulnerable person that has occurred as a result of health- and social-care professionals not collaborating effectively.

There can be no doubt that interprofessional working can improve patient outcome, but change is uncomfortable and health- and social-care professionals are currently experiencing rapid and significant changes to both their working practices and to the environment within which they are working. This process of change will need to be carefully and sensitively managed if we are to achieve effective interprofessional working with an integrated patient-focused service.

Against this backdrop, this book is designed to provide you with the underpinning theoretical knowledge, understanding and skills to work effectively as a member of an interprofessional team. The book offers you practical advice and tips to help guide your practice to work and learn within an interprofessional context. There are two principal underpinning narrative threads:

- The developments in UK health- and social-care policy that have positioned interprofessional working at the centre of contemporary health- and social-care systems.

- The importance of ensuring that patients are the focus of care and that all health- and social-care professionals work as an integrated team to provide quality care in the best interests of the patient.

Each chapter explores a different aspect of interprofessional working. Chapter 1 uses an interprofessional practice-based scenario to introduce you to all the different aspects of interprofessional working. It also explores the semantic quagmire related to the term 'interprofessional'. In Chapter 2 we explore the context of inter-professional working and you will be introduced to all the relevant UK health- and social-care policies and legislation that are impacting on interprofessional developments in practice. Subsequent chapters deal with teams, team work and team dynamics; expertise and leadership; communicating with each other; learning within an interprofessional environment; and interprofessional learning within a practice environment. The final chapter of the book identifies the barriers to effective interprofessional working and offers practical suggestions for overcoming these barriers.

Within health and social care, various terms are used to refer to the person receiving care including patient, client and service user. For the sake of simplicity, in this book, the term patient will be used throughout.

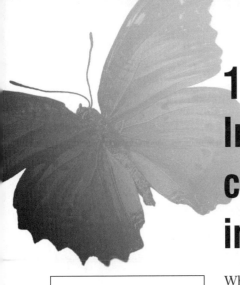

1

Introduction – The key concepts of interprofessional working

Learning outcomes

By the end of this chapter you should be able to:

★ Identify the key concepts of effective interprofessional working

★ Explain the term 'interprofessional'

★ Be aware of the different organisational levels at which health- and social-care professionals are required to work together to provide effective delivery of care to the patient and their family and carers.

When you are working and learning within the health- or social-care setting, hardly a day goes by without you hearing terms such as: interprofessional; partnership; collaboration; teamwork; patient-focused care; seamless care; interagency. But what do all these terms mean and why is working and learning together so important? Where does the patient fit in and what does it all mean for the patient?

Interprofessional working, or simply working and learning together, is recognised by health- and social-care professionals, patients and their carers, health- and social-care educationalists and policy makers as a 'good' thing and a 'worthwhile and achievable ambition'. Over the last 10 years, significant progress has been made towards creating the necessary environment within which interprofessional working can flourish. People are no longer questioning whether interprofessional working is important but have progressed to focusing on how best to make it work.

It has been suggested that health- and social-care professionals are required to work together at three different levels (Department of Health, 1998a):

1. At a **strategic** level, agencies are required to plan together and share information about the use of their resources.

2. At the level of **operational management**, a range of policies are required that demonstrate partnership.

3. At the level of **individual care and support**, for example, people expect a single point of access into the health care system, shared information systems for interprofessional teams, and joint training.

So how do we make interprofessional working happen effectively at these three levels? This book is designed to provide you with the necessary skills and theoretical knowledge and understanding to practise effectively within an interprofessional team. Included within the book are practical suggestions and advice on all aspects of interprofessional working.

In this introductory chapter, we will use a case study to highlight the key concepts of interprofessional working that will be presented in the following chapters. This will be followed by a discussion that unpicks the terminology used within the context of working and learning together.

Interprofessional working and the delivery of effective care

Mrs Jones is a 62-year-old widow who enters hospital for a planned below-the-knee amputation as a result of diabetic foot ulceration. She lives alone in a two-storey house, with a bedroom and bathroom upstairs. Her only daughter lives locally and she has no other family. Mrs Jones has a cat and dog to whom she is devoted. When Mrs Jones is admitted to hospital, her immediate neighbour looks after her cat and dog. She has a very good friend, who gives her a lift to the hospital for her appointments. Hospital transport has been offered to Mrs Jones but she does not like waiting.

Mrs Jones is a heavy smoker and smokes at least 20–30 cigarettes a day. She also enjoys her food, although she is not overweight. She refuses to compromise on either cigarettes or food as she feels these are some of the few pleasures left in her life.

Box 1.1

There would appear to be an opportunity for health care professionals to promote a healthier lifestyle for Mrs Jones. Recent government policies and initiatives have focused on improving the health of the individual, and thus the population as a whole, with the emphasis being on preventative care. Mrs Jones smokes heavily. All those professionals caring for her have a responsibility to advise her to stop smoking and offer her the necessary support should she wish to stop. Smoking cessation services are a key part of the government's NHS modernisation agenda. The following government documents give a central place to smoking cessation services: the White Paper, *Smoking Kills* (Department of Health, 1998b); *The NHS Plan* (Department of Health, 2000a); *The Cancer Plan* (Department of Health, 2000b); the *National Service Framework for Coronary Heart Disease* (Department of Health, 2000c); and the *NHS Smoking Cessation Services* (Department of Health, 2001a). In Chapter 2 we will explore the health- and social-care policies and legislation which have encouraged interprofessional working and patient-centred care.

Mrs Jones has had Type 2 diabetes mellitus for 25 years, which is tablet controlled. However, her management of her diabetes is poor, which has resulted in her having had a stroke several years ago. The stroke affected her speech and impaired her mobility. Mrs Jones' mobility was already limited due to the ulceration of her foot. She uses a Zimmer frame to help her mobility. Her neighbour does her shopping for her, as Mrs Jones rarely leaves her house.

Box 1.2

Mrs Jones does not manage her diabetes very well. She could take advantage of, and may benefit from, attending a DESMOND (Diabetes Education and Self-Management for Ongoing and Newly Diagnosed) programme. This is a structured patient education programme for people with Type 2 diabetes.

continued

continued

One of the key drivers for setting up this national programme was to meet Standard 3 of the *National Service Framework for Diabetes* (Department of Health, 2001b). NSFs were one of the developments that arose from the White Paper, *A First Class Service: Quality in the New NHS* (Department of Health, 1998a).

To support the development of structured education for people with diabetes, an interprofessional Diabetes UK Patient Education Working Group was set up in 2004. This group worked with the Department of Health and published the document, *Structured Patient Education in Diabetes* (Department of Health, 2005). The DESMOND education programme was one of the national programmes that resulted from this publication. This is another example of how health- and social-care policies have encouraged interprofessional working and patient-centred care.

Mrs Jones has required previous hospital admissions for diabetic foot ulceration. These have been over a long period of time, which has resulted in Mrs Jones forming a dislike of all medical, nursing and physiotherapy staff. Mrs Jones is a very independent lady and her admissions to hospital have made her realise that, due to her condition, she is gradually losing her independence. She believes that the goalposts are moved by those health professionals caring for her and is, therefore, cynical about what they are telling her.

However, there are a few members of the interprofessional team that Mrs Jones does bond well with and she will communicate with these members of staff. These health care professionals are the diabetes nurse specialist, Susan, and one of her consultants, Dr Melson. Mrs Jones likes these two because they are straight talking and the language they use is easy to understand.

Keywords

Angiogram

An X-ray diagnostic procedure used to visualise the blood vessels following injection of a contrast substance into an artery. An angiogram is used to image arteries in the brain, heart, kidneys, gastrointestinal tract, aorta, neck, chest, limbs and pulmonary circuit

Angioplasty

The surgical repair of a blood vessel. A balloon angioplasty is a non-invasive procedure where a balloon-tipped catheter is introduced into a diseased blood vessel. As the balloon is inflated, the vessel opens allowing an improved flow of blood

Box 1.3

Mrs Jones has indicated that she finds it difficult to understand all of the information being communicated to her by the health care professionals caring for her. Effective communication between health- and social-care professional and patient is considered essential for effective interprofessional working and the consequent delivery of quality health- and social-care to patients. Professional language and jargon are often cited as a barrier to effective communication and therefore to interprofessional working. In Chapter 7, we will identify the barriers to effective interprofessional working and look at the impact that such barriers have on providing effective health- and social-care delivery.

Mrs Jones presents to the diabetic centre with an extensive ulcer in the region of her ankle, which has been non-healing for a number of months. The topical treatments that have been prescribed are not working. She is reviewed at the foot clinic, within the diabetes centre, and is seen jointly by her consultant, Susan (the diabetes nurse specialist) and a podiatrist (the diabetes team). Following the consultation, the diabetes team decide to offer Mrs Jones an **angiogram/angioplasty**. As Mrs Jones trusts Susan, it is Susan who discusses the preferred treatment option with her. At first, Mrs Jones refuses to be admitted to hospital because it is close to Christmas. Eventually, she agrees to be admitted to hospital after Christmas.

continued

Box 1.4

The diabetic team are all experts in their field. The consultant, diabetes nurse specialist and the podiatrist all contribute different but complementary knowledge, skills and expertise to the care of Mrs Jones. Each member of the team is aware of the roles and responsibilities of the others. In this case study, Susan, the diabetic nurse specialist, demonstrates some of the key characteristics of an expert: she is knowledgeable; she excels in her own domain; she values the participation of the consultant, podiatrist and district nurse in the decision-making process; and she is patient-centred in her approach.

It appears from the above that the diabetic team work well together and that, depending on the circumstance, different team members can take the lead. There appears to be a horizontal team structure as opposed to the traditional hierarchical team structure. In Chapter 4, Leadership and Expertise, we will discuss effective leadership; consider the complex nature of expertise and look at how expertise influences the leadership within an interprofessional team.

While Mrs Jones is waiting to be admitted, the district nurse continues to visit her on a daily basis, to clean and dress her ulcer. Mrs Jones has a 'communication book', which she takes with her to the diabetic centre. This book helps Susan to communicate with the district nurse who is caring for Mrs Jones on a daily basis.

Box 1.5

Mrs Jones' care is being shared between primary and secondary care teams. The majority of her care is provided within secondary (specialist) care, liaising with primary care. As we can see from this case study, the professionals in her primary care team include her GP; pharmacist; and district nurse. The professionals in her secondary care team include her consultant (with specialist training in diabetes), a podiatrist and a diabetes nurse specialist. The 'communication book' is one method of communication used by the primary and secondary care teams. Mrs Jones keeps the book, and she takes it to all her appointments at the diabetic clinic. The diabetes nurse specialist can write down suggestions on how to treat Mrs Jones' diabetic ulcer. The district nurse is then able to implement the suggestions made by the diabetes nurse specialist and can write in the book whether they worked or not. This is one method of communication and can enhance the effectiveness of teamwork. The district nurse and the diabetic nurse specialist will also communicate verbally, using the telephone. In Chapter 3 we will consider the different types of team, identify what helps and hinders effective teamwork and discuss the benefits of working in a team.

Mrs Jones is admitted to hospital after Christmas and attends the radiology department for her angiogram. Susan is in attendance to provide moral support for Mrs Jones. During this investigation, Mrs Jones is uncommunicative with the staff in the radiology department, who have to rely on Susan for information. Susan believes that Mrs Jones is not communicating because she is scared about undergoing the investigation and is also afraid of the outcome of the angiogram.

Unfortunately, the result from the angiogram is not good. The diabetes team meet to discuss the preferred management option for Mrs Jones following the results. Mrs Jones is informed of the decision during a ward round. In attendance are her consultant, senior house officers, a nurse from the ward and Susan. The consultant explains to Mrs Jones that she will need to have a below-the-knee amputation. Mrs Jones does not ask any questions of any of the health care professionals in attendance. After the consultant has left, Susan explains the procedure to Mrs Jones, on a one-to-one basis. Mrs Jones communicates with Susan in a very matter-of-fact manner but it is obviously difficult for her to come to terms with losing part of her leg.

Following the operation, Mrs Jones' amputation heals well and there are no complications. Susan visits her on the ward on a daily basis to provide emotional support and discusses with Mrs Jones the practicalities of going home and living alone in her two-storey home.

The physiotherapist also visits Mrs Jones on a daily basis. Mrs Jones finds it difficult to get on with her physiotherapist, David, as she thinks that he does not understand how much her stroke is affecting her ability to mobilise.

The ward staff inform Susan, during one of her visits to the ward, that Mrs Jones has been abrupt and uncooperative. Mrs Jones believes that the ward staff have little insight into her situation. At this point Mrs Jones becomes very tearful, which improves the situation as it makes the ward staff realise that much of her perceived abruptness is purely a defence mechanism and it also allows Mrs Jones to see how supportive the ward staff are. Trips away from the ward with Susan appear to ease the tension. Going to the café provides the opportunity for Susan to chat with Mrs Jones in a relaxed environment. It is clear to Susan that Mrs Jones is very anxious to go home.

Box 1.6

As we have seen in this case study, Mrs Jones' previous experiences of attending hospital have not been positive and this has resulted in her finding it difficult to communicate with the health- and social-care professionals caring for her. Despite this, it is clear that all the professionals involved in her care communicate with her and try to involve her in the planning of her care and treatment. Susan, her diabetic nurse specialist, is a key health professional in Mrs Jones' care and, as we have seen, it is often Susan who communicates with the other health- and social-care professionals on her behalf. It is clear from the case study that the health- and social-care professionals involved in Mrs Jones' care and treatment liaise effectively with each other and that her pathway through the health- and social-care system is smooth and efficient.

In Chapter 5 we will explore the methods of communication which enhance effective interprofessional working, discuss the fundamental communication skills needed to facilitate effective relationships with service users and health care professionals and discuss the barriers to effective communication.

Six weeks after her operation, a home assessment is arranged for Mrs Jones by an occupational therapist. Mrs Jones and the occupational therapist visit her home together and assess what adaptations need to be in place before she can be discharged home permanently. The adaptations required are minimal: her bed needs to be brought downstairs and a commode is necessary. However, leading up to Mrs Jones' front door is a very high step, which means that once in the house she

continued

cannot get out again. Mrs Jones is adamant that she wants to go home. It is agreed that she can be discharged provided that this is not a long-term solution and that more suitable accommodation is found very quickly.

Before Mrs Jones is discharged, she meets with a member of social services to start the process of finding alternative accommodation. Mrs Jones is discharged two weeks later and moves into a bungalow not long after going home.

Box 1.7

This case ends on a positive note, with Mrs Jones leaving hospital happy and with everything in place for her independent living. Her final contact with health care professionals is a positive one, which should mean that she will not be reluctant to come back into hospital should she need to.

An effective interprofessional team is evident in this case study and an integrated care package individualised for Mrs Jones has been provided. This case study demonstrates what can be achieved if health- and social-care professionals are working collaboratively with a patient-centred approach. In Chapter 6 we will consider the importance of interprofessional learning and look at ways in which a learning environment where effective interprofessional learning can take place can be created.

With reference to the case study:

- Draw a diagram to show the health- and social-care professionals who came into contact with Mrs Jones before she was admitted to hospital, while she was in hospital and after she was discharged.
- Consider how important the role of the diabetes nurse specialist was in providing care and support for Mrs Jones.
- How could the communication between Mrs Jones and the professionals caring for her have been enhanced?
- What further support could have been provided for Mrs Jones either before, during or after her stay in hospital?

What does the term 'interprofessional' mean?

At first this might seem like a straightforward question that would have a very straightforward unequivocal answer. However, this is not the case, with the literature revealing that the term 'interprofessional' is not a clearly defined concept, resulting in what Leathard (1994, p. 5) refers to as a 'terminological quagmire'. In this section we will attempt to unravel this 'terminological quagmire' and identify the working definitions that will be used in this book.

Reflective activity

There are a range of terms that are used interchangeably to suggest interprofessional working. List all the terms that you have come across that refer to people working and learning together.

Leathard (1994, p. 5) identified a number of terms that have been used to indicate working and learning together and categorised them into three groups:

1. **Concept based** – for example, interdisciplinary, interprofessional, multidisciplinary, multiprofessional.
2. **Process based** – for example, joint planning, joint training, teamwork, partnership, collaboration, cooperation, coordination, participation, collaborative working, joint working, joint learning.
3. **Agency based** – for example, interagency, inter-sectoral, trans-sectoral, consortium, alliance.

Rawson (1994, p. 39) uses an alternative grouping of terms, based on three sets of concepts:

1. **Problematic association**: inter/multi/trans
2. **Grouping**: professional/occupational/disciplinary/sectoral/ agency
3. **Focus of operations**: work/teamwork/collaboration/ cooperation/integration.

Barr (2002, p. 30) groups the terms according to whether they are prefixes, adjectives or nouns:

1. **Prefixes**: inter/multi/trans/cross
2. **Adjectives**: professional/disciplinary
3. **Nouns**: education/training/studies/learning.

All these terms can and have been put together in what appears to be endless permutations, all of which signify working and learning together. We need to clarify this 'terminological quagmire' before we move on and explore interprofessional working within the UK context.

We will begin the process of clarification by defining each individual term, using the categorisation put forward by Rawson (1994). Once each individual term has been defined, we will then combine terms and explore what the terms mean when related to learning and working together. This will provide a shared understanding of these terms that will help you understand the context within which this book refers to interprofessional working.

The first category we will consider is 'problem association'.

- **Inter**: 'between, among; mutually; reciprocally' (*Compact Oxford English Dictionary*, 2005).

  'denotes relationships both between and among the elements and further implies some notion of reciprocal operations' (Rawson, 1994, p. 40)

- **Multi**: 'more than one, many' (*Compact Oxford English Dictionary*, 2005).

  'implies many and some form of composition but . . . does not immediately suggest any give and take [within the group]' (Rawson, 1994, p. 40)

- **Trans**: 'across, beyond; on or to the other side of' (*Compact Oxford English Dictionary*, 2005).

  'signifies relationships across or beyond but does not carry any indication of mutuality' (Rawson, 1994, p. 40).

Next we will consider the terms within the category 'grouping':

- **Professional**: 'relating to or belonging to a profession' (*Compact Oxford English Dictionary*, 2005).

  Being a professional person is associated with particular distinctive features, which include:

  - membership of a restricted and regulated professional association, for example, Nursing and Midwifery Council (NMC), Health Professions Council (HPC)
  - having a great deal of autonomy
  - mastery of a specific body of knowledge, skills and expertise
  - an extensive period of education and training prior to practising
  - a philosophy of public service and altruism.

  Historically there were only three professions: medical doctors, lawyers and clergy. Professions such as nursing and social work were classified as semi-professions because of perceived limitations to their knowledge base, training and autonomy (Etzioni, 1969)

- **Occupational**: This is a broader term than 'professional', which leaves out the strong identity denoted by the term 'professional'

- **Disciplinary**: The noun 'discipline' is defined as 'a branch of knowledge, especially one studied in higher education' (*Compact Oxford English Dictionary*, 2005).

  The term 'disciplinary' suggests a narrower term than professional

- **Sectoral**: The noun 'sector' refers to 'an area or portion that is distinct from others, a distinct part of an economy, society or sphere of activity' (*Compact Oxford English Dictionary*, 2005).

  'Sectoral' refers to an organisational feature rather than a group of people

- **Agency**: 'an organisation providing a particular service; a government office or department providing a specific service' (*Compact Oxford English Dictionary*, 2005).

  'Agency', like 'sectoral', is referring to an organisational feature. It is a narrower term than 'sectoral', and its definition implies that there may be a number of agencies within a sector.

Finally we will consider the third of Rawson's (1994) categories, focus of operations.

- **Collaboration**: 'work jointly on an activity or project' (*Compact Oxford English Dictionary*, 2005).

  'Collaboration' describes working together to achieve something that neither agency could achieve alone (Biggs, 1997, p. 188)

- **Cooperation**: 'work jointly towards the same end' (*Compact Oxford English Dictionary*, 2005).

  'Cooperation' implies 'working together with positive connotations' (Biggs, 1997, p. 188)

- **Teamwork**: 'Teamwork is the way people work together cooperatively and effectively' (Manion *et al.* 1996).

Having defined the individual terms we will combine some of them in an attempt to determine the definition we will use in this book to embody working and learning together.

Firstly, we will consider 'interprofessional' which is, of course, in the title of this book. If we put the definitions of 'inter' and 'professional' together we would come up with a definition such as the following:

> Persons belonging to a profession, relating between and among each other, for the mutual benefit of those involved.

This definition implies that if the different professional groups relate with each other there will be a synergist effect and that more will be achieved by the different groups relating with each other than if they were not. It must also be remembered that within any one workplace, the interprofessional relations need to take into account that there will be different professional groups working within the same organisation and that the same professional groups will be working across different organisations. This begins to build up a picture of the complexity we are dealing with when we start to explore interprofessional working and learning.

However, before accepting this definition there needs to be further clarification of the term 'professional'. As noted earlier, historically there were only three professions, with others classed as semi-professions. If you continue to use such a restrictive definition of a profession, this will mean certain key groups will be excluded, for example police, teachers, patients and their carers, voluntary workers, leisure staff. All of these groups are important in the context of the wellbeing of people and therefore you would wish the term used to denote working and learning together to be an inclusive term. I would suggest, therefore, that within this book we use a less literal definition of a profession, to enable all groups that are working and learning together to provide health- and social-care for patients to be included within the term.

Combining 'inter' and 'professional' has combined two out of three of Rawson's (1994) categories. If we combine 'interprofessional' with terms from Rawson's (1994) third category 'focus of operations' we create terms such as:

- interprofessional learning
- interprofessional education
- interprofessional collaboration
- interprofessional teamwork.

All of these terms can be found within the literature. To work out the meaning of each term, you simply take the definition of 'interprofessional' and add it to the definition of the term from the third category, that is, collaboration, teamwork, education and learning.

Probably one of the most frequently used and widely accepted definitions of interprofessional education is that proposed by the Centre for the Advancement of Interprofessional Education (CAIPE, 1997):

> Occasions when two or more professions learn from and about each other to improve collaboration and the quality of care.

In this book, when referring to interprofessional education, we will be using this definition.

The next term that is frequently used within the literature is 'multiprofessional'. If we put together the definitions of 'multi' and 'professional', we would come up with a definition such as the following:

> Professionals from more than one/many professions coming together but not necessarily for the mutual benefit of the professionals involved.

The fundamental difference between 'multiprofessional' and 'interprofessional' is that multiprofessional activities bring two or more groups of professionals together to work on a specific task, but there is little collaboration. The different professional groups bring different professional perspectives to the task, but there is no sense of this being done to gain a synergistic effect, that is, to develop a perspective that is more than the sum of the individual parts. In multiprofessional activities, those participating gain an understanding of their separate but interrelated roles (Pirrie *et al.*, 1998).

If we then combine the term 'multiprofessional' with Rawson's (1994) third category, 'focus of operations', we create the following terms which can be frequently found within the literature:

- multiprofessional education
- multiprofessional working.

CAIPE (1997), as well as defining interprofessional education, have also defined multiprofessional education:

> Occasions when two or more professions learn side by side for whatever reason.

The terms 'interprofessional' and 'multiprofessional' are those that tend to be used most frequently within the literature. There are, however, many others that can be found and different organisations and groups tend to favour particular forms. Policy makers, for example, prefer to use terms such as joint training; partnership working; joint working; interagency. In this book, therefore, when discussing health- and social-care policies and legislation, these terms will be used.

Academics tend to prefer terms such as 'interprofessional', 'multiprofessional', 'interdisciplinary' and 'multidisciplinary'. Some universities prefer the term 'multiprofessional education' as this is the preferred term of the World Health Organization (WHO, 1988).

Different professions use language very differently, which means they may interpret very differently the terms we have just defined. Pietroni (1992) identified 11 distinct language subsets used by health- and social-care professionals. This illustrates the potential for different interpretations to exist between the different professional groups.

RRRR*Rapid recap*

Check your progress so far by working through each of the following questions.

1. What are the three levels that health- and social-care professionals need to work together at if interprofessional working is to be successful?
2. What is the difference between interprofessional working and multiprofessional working?

3. What is interprofessional education?
4. What is interagency working?

If you have difficulty with more than one of the questions, read through the section again to refresh your understanding before moving on.

References

Barr, H. (2002) Interprofessional Education: Today, Yesterday and Tomorrow. Learning and Teaching Support Network for Health Sciences and Practice, London. Available from: www.health.heacademy.co.uk.

Biggs, S. (1997) Interprofessional Collaboration: Problems and Prospects' In Øvretveit, J., Mathias, P. and Thomson, T. (eds.). *Interprofessional Working for Health- and social-care*. Macmillan, London, pp. 186–200.

CAIPE (1997) Interprofessional Education – A Definition. *CAIPE Bulletin*, No. 13.

Department of Health (1998a) *Partnership in Action (New Opportunities for Joint Working Between Health and Social Services)* Department of Health, London. Available from: www.dh.gov.uk.

Department of Health (1998b) *Smoking Kills. A White Paper on Tobacco*. The Stationery Office, London.

Department of Health (1998c) *A First Class Service: Quality in the New NHS*. HMSO, London. Available from: www.dh.gov.uk.

Department of Health (2000a) *The NHS Plan: A Plan for Investment, a Plan for Reform*. London: HMSO Available from: www.dh.gov.uk.

Department of Health (2000b) *The NHS Cancer Plan*. HMSO, London. Available from: www.dh.gov.uk.

Department of Health (2000c) *National Service Framework for Coronary Heart Disease*. HMSO, London. Available from: www.dh.gov.uk.

Department of Health (2001a) *NHS Smoking Cessation Services. Service and Monitoring Guidance 2001/02*. HMSO, London.

Department of Health (2001b) *National Service Framework for Diabetes*. HMSO, London. Available from: www.dh.gov.uk.

Department of Health (2005) *Structured Patient Education in Diabetes*. HMSO, London. Available from: www.dh.gov.uk.

Etzioni, A. (ed.) (1969) *The Semi-professions and their Organisation*. Free Press, Macmillan, New York.

Leathard, A. (1994) Interprofessional Developments in Britain: an Overview. In *Going Interprofessional: Working Together for Health and Welfare* (ed. Leathard, A.). Routledge, London, pp. 3–37

Manion, J., Lorimer, W. and Leander, W.J. (1996) *Team-based Health Care Organisations: Blueprint for Success*. Apsen, Gaithersburg, MD.

Murray, J.A.H., Simpson, J. and Weiner, E. (eds.) (2005) *The Compact Oxford English Dictionary*. Oxford English Press, Oxford.

Pietroni, P.C. (1992) Towards Reflective Practice – The Language of Health- and Social-care. *Journal of Interprofessional Care*, **6**: 7–16.

Pirrie, A., Wilson, V., Elsegood, J., Hall, J., Hamilton, S., Harden, R., Lee, D. and Stead, J. (1998) *Evaluating Multidisciplinary Education in Health Care*. SCRE, Edinburgh.

Rawson, D. (1994) Models of Interprofessional Work: Likely Theories and Possibilities. In *Going Interprofessional: Working Together for Health and Welfare* (ed. Leathard, A.). Routledge, London, pp. 38–63.

World Health Organization (1988) *Learning Together to Work Together for Health*. WHO, Geneva.

2
The context of interprofessional working

Learning outcomes

By the end of this chapter you should be able to:

★ Identify the relevant UK health- and social-care policies and legislation that are impacting on interprofessional developments in practice

★ Understand the importance of participating effectively in interprofessional and multi-agency approaches to the delivery of health- and social care

★ Be aware of the historical circumstances that initiated the recent interprofessional developments.

Historical overview of interprofessional developments

In this section we will trace the development of interprofessional working from when the National Health Service was first set up in 1948 through to the present day. There has been a plethora of health- and social-care policies and legislation published in the UK, which has helped to shape interprofessional working. For simplicity's sake, therefore, only the key health- and social-care policies and legislation will be highlighted and discussed.

Interprofessional working is not a new concept. The history of health- and social care is full of calls for the different professions and the agencies to collaborate. In fact, the value of collaboration between health, social care and employment was recognised as far back as The Beveridge Report in 1942. Despite this report, however, the National Health Act 1946 and the National Assistance Act 1948 created a system whereby health- and social care were separated rather than being brought together (Hugman, 1995). Thus, collaboration between health- and social-care professionals and between health- and social-care services were made more difficult in 1948 when the National Health Service was formed.

It is important to remember that for the development of collaboration and effective interprofessional working, not only do the health- and social-care professionals need to want to collaborate, but also the organisational structures need to be in place for this to be possible. Health- and social-care policies , therefore, do not only need to encourage professionals to work together but also need to put the appropriate organisational structures in place.

Key UK health- and social-care reports, policies and legislation

The Seebohm Report, 1968

This report identified that closer working relationships between social services and general practitioners (GPs) was desirable, stating:

> Survey after survey has shown that many family doctors do not seek help from social workers nor use social services that are available, they often do not know about them, or do not understand or value them . . . Realistic attempts at prevention in the social field whether in detecting early trouble or intervening at times of crisis . . . will often have to be based on family practice and organised as a joint effort of doctors and social workers.
>
> (Seebohm Report 1968, para. 692, cited in Lymbery, 1998)

The Seebohm Report was published almost 40 years ago and 40 years on we are still hearing calls for health- and social-care professionals to develop more effective collaborative working.

The Alma Ata Declaration (World Health Organization, 1978)

The Alma Ata Declaration was defined following a World Health Organization conference on primary health care held in Alma Ata in the former USSR. The declaration called for a more holistic approach to primary care to be taken, with the establishment of community health centres and community health workers.

This declaration placed the patient and their family and carers at the centre of their care, encouraging them to fully participate in the discussions and decisions made about care and treatment, that is, a patient-focused care approach was being advocated.

Working for Patients (Department of Health, 1989a)

This White Paper outlined the most significant cultural shift that the NHS had seen since its inception in 1948, with the introduction of the internal market. The internal market gave 'purchasers' (health authorities and some GPs) budgets to buy health care from 'providers' (acute hospitals; organisations providing care for the mentally ill, the elderly, people with learning disabilities; and ambulance services). To become a 'provider', health organisations became NHS Trusts, independent organisations with their own managements, competing with each other. The aims of this White Paper included:

- to make the health service more responsive to the needs of patients
- to devolve as much responsibility to local level as possible
- to allow the money needed to treat patients to cross administrative boundaries
- to allow large GP practices to hold their own budgets.

This White Paper began to make the organisational changes that were required to make interprofessional working possible.

Caring for People: Community Care in the Next Decade and Beyond (Department of Health, 1989b)

This White Paper described how local authority social services departments organise and provide community care services. Its overall aim was to promote a range of community care services to enable vulnerable people to live in the community whenever possible.

The NHS and Community Care Act 1990

The NHS and Community Care Act 1990 made the legal changes necessary for the new arrangements set out in the White Papers, *Working for Patients* (Department of Health, 1989a) and *Caring for People: Community Care in the Next Decade and Beyond* (1989b).

The New NHS, Modern – Dependable (Secretary of State for Health, 1997)

This White Paper signalled the biggest programme of change the NHS had seen since its inception in 1948. Following the election of a new government in 1997, Tony Blair declared that the publication of this White Paper was to be a turning point for the NHS and was the start of a process of modernisation.

After 50 years of policies and legislation designed to encourage health- and social-care professionals to work with each other and across services and agencies, including the voluntary and private sector, this White Paper provided the necessary impetus for interprofessional working to become a reality.

The White Paper announced an end to the inequities and inefficiencies of the internal market, replacing it with a system of integrated care based on partnership and driven by performance. To facilitate the development of integrated care, the White Paper reported that organisational barriers would be broken down and that patients would no longer be passed back and forth between different agencies with competing agendas. The claim was that cooperation would replace competition and that the NHS would forge new working relationships locally with education, employment, housing and social services.

This White Paper was essentially about putting patients at the heart of the NHS and moving the focus from a service that does things to and for its patients to one that works with patients.

This new approach to the NHS was based on six key principles:

- to renew the NHS as a genuinely national service
- to make the delivery of health care against those new national standards a matter of local responsibility
- to get the NHS to work in partnership, breaking down organisational barriers and forging stronger links with local authorities
- to improve efficiency so that every pound in the NHS is spent to maximise the care for patients

- to shift the focus onto quality of care so that excellence is guaranteed to all patients
- to rebuild public confidence in the NHS.

If we review this White Paper, we can see that three main themes emerge:

1. partnership working
2. patient-centred care
3. organisational changes to make themes one and two possible.

Thus, in 1997, new ways of working and collaboration on a scale not previously seen within the NHS began to be introduced.

Health- and social-care policies since the publication of *The New NHS, Modern – Dependable* (Secretary of State for Health, 1997) have set out the changes which need to be made within the NHS and social services in order to implement the vision laid out within this White Paper.

Modernising Social Services (Department of Health, 1998a)

In this White Paper specific mention was made to the problems within social services and why modernisation was necessary. The problems highlighted included:

- lack of safeguards to protect vulnerable children and adults
- lack of coordination of services
- inflexibility
- lack of clarity of role
- lack of consistency
- inefficiency.

Improving partnerships was one of the ways in which these problems were to be tackled, with the White Paper stating:

> We are legislating to improve joint working between health and social services. This will allow for pooling of budgets and other ways to deliver truly integrated care that is geared to the needs of individuals. We are also improving partnership with housing and other services, and introducing stronger children's services planning requirements to ensure more effective co-ordination of services for children.

This White Paper clearly demonstrates the three main themes, that is, partnership, patient-centred care and organisational change, that were identified in the White Paper, *The New NHS, Modern – Dependable* (Secretary of State for Health, 1997) as being essential for the modernisation of the NHS.

Modernising Government (National Audit Office, 1999)

This White Paper was central to the government's programme of modernisation. Within this White Paper a commitment was made to:

- ensuring that policy making was more joined up and strategic
- delivering public services to meet the needs of citizens, not the convenience of service providers
- delivering a big push on obstacles to joined-up working, through local partnerships, one-stop shops and other means.

Modernising Government (National Audit Offic, 1999) primarily focuses on the organisational changes that are necessary for effective interprofessional working.

National Service Frameworks (NSFs) 1999–2005

The NSFs were one of the developments that arose from the White Paper, *A First Class Service: Quality in the New NHS* (Department of Health, 1998b). The NSFs cover the highest-priority conditions in the UK – cancer and coronary heart disease, other common conditions including diabetes and mental health and some of the key patient groups – children and older people. NSFs have two main roles, they:

- set clear quality requirements for care, based on the best available evidence of what treatments and services work effectively for patients
- offer strategies and support to help organisations achieve these.

One strength of the NSFs is that they were developed in partnership with health professionals, patients, carers, health-service managers, voluntary agencies and other experts. Partnership is a key theme within all the NSFs. For example, *National Service Framework for Older People* (Department of Health, 2001a) advocated a single assessment process. The need for each health- and social-care professional to undertake their own assessment of an older person was no longer required. This means that a single, tailored care package can be developed for the older person and be delivered by specialist networks of professionals working across primary, community and hospital settings. The children's NSF (Department of Health, 2004a) aimed to ensure that the care the child and their parents and/or carers receive is better coordinated, so that they do not have to see too many professionals and repeat their story over and over again.

The Health Act 1999 – Modern Partnerships for People (Department of Health, 1999a)

The Health Act 1999 provided new powers to enable health and local authority partners to work together more effectively. These new powers were referred to as flexibilities. The purpose of the flexibilities was to enable partners, for example health bodies (Primary Care Trusts,

Strategic Health Authorities) and any health-related local authority services (social services, community and acute services, housing) to join together to design and deliver services around the needs of the patient rather than worrying about the boundaries of their organisations. These arrangements were designed to eliminate unnecessary gaps and duplications between services.

The new powers/flexibilities were:

- pooled funds – the partners were able to each contribute agreed funds to a single pot, to be spent on agreed projects for designated services
- lead commissioning – the partners were able to delegate commissioning of a service to one lead organisation
- integrated provision – the partners were able to combine their staff, resources and management structures to integrate the provision of a service from managerial level to the front line.

Agenda for Change: Modernising the NHS Pay System
(Department of Health, 1999b)

Differences in payment, conditions of service and rewards have been cited as a barrier to interprofessional working (Headrick *et al.*, 1998). *Agenda for Change* was a radical change to the pay system for all staff directly employed by the NHS, with the exception of very senior managers and those covered by the Doctors' and Dentists' Pay Review Body. The new pay system was designed to overcome the barriers identified by Headrick *et al.* (1998).

There are three elements to *Agenda for Change*:

1. The new terms and conditions of employment
2. The *Agenda for Change* pay and band structure underpinned by the NHS job evaluation scheme
3. The *NHS Knowledge and Skills Framework* (Department of Health, 2003).

The new NHS pay system is based on the principle of equal pay for work of equal value and will provide:

- greater scope to create new kinds of jobs, bringing more patient-centred care and more varied and stimulating roles for NHS staff
- a fair and transparent pay system based on on-the-job evaluation
- harmonisation of conditions of service, for example working hours
- links between pay, skills and knowledge
- greater support for team working through harmonised, out-of-hours and overtime arrangements.

This new pay system was introduced in 12 'early implementer' sites in 2003 and the process of implementation across the entire NHS began in 2004 and was completed in 2006.

The NHS Plan: a plan for investment, a plan for reform (Department of Health, 2000a)

It was not until *The NHS Plan* was published in 2000 that the plans to transform the NHS as described in the White Paper, *The New NHS, Modern – Dependable* (Secretary of State for Health, 1997) came into focus. This White Paper described a 10-year plan that was designed to tackle the systemic problems of the NHS which dated from when it was formed in 1948. These systemic problems included:

- old-fashioned demarcations between staff and barriers between services
- over-centralised and disempowered patients
- a lack of standards
- a lack of clear incentives and levers to improve performance.

Reforms included within *The NHS Plan* designed to enhance interprofessional working included:

- Care Trusts were created to provide better-integrated health- and social care. Care Trusts, an NHS body, are designed to bring the NHS responsibilities and local authority health responsibilities together under a single management structure. This structural change in health- and social-care provision should increase continuity of care and simplify administration. Care Trusts were introduced in 2002.

- Nurses and other staff are to have a greater opportunity to extend their roles. This reform was designed to develop a flexible work-force, where multiple professionals are able to take on tasks traditionally seen as the domain of one profession. Since the publication of *The NHS Plan*, there have been a host of new roles created, including assistant practitioners; advanced practitioners; non-medical consultants, in, for example, radiography, nursing, midwifery and health visiting; non-medical prescribing for nurses and allied health professionals; community matrons and modern matrons.

The Health- and Social-Care Act 2001 (Department of Health, 2001b)

This Act was the legislation that allowed the reforms outlined in *The NHS Plan* (Department of Health, 2000) to be taken forward. The Act covered a range of measures related to primary care, long-term care of the elderly, patient advocacy, nurse prescribing and the creation of Care Trusts.

Knowledge and Skills Framework (KSF) (Department of Health, 2003)

The NHS KSF was introduced under *Agenda for Change* (Department of Health, 1999b) and is central to the learning and development, career and pay progressions elements of *Agenda for Change*. The NHS KSF is a broad, generic framework that sets out to describe and recognise the types of knowledge and skills that a post holder needs to be effective in their NHS job.

Under *Agenda for Change* all staff are entitled to an annual review. During this annual review a personal development plan will be prepared. The KSF is designed to provide a fair and objective framework on which to base this annual review and development of staff.

Using the NHS KSF will enable team leaders to identify gaps in the knowledge and skills of their interprofessional team. This will facilitate the development of an annual team staff development plan.

Evidence base

Go to the website www.dh.gov.uk and read the *The NHS Knowledge and Skills Framework* (NHS KSF) and the *Development Review Process* (October 2004).

The NHS Improvement Plan: Putting People at the Heart of Public Services (Department of Health, 2004b)

In this publication, the Department of Health once again pledged their commitment to greater flexibility and growth in the way services are provided, which will be matched by increases in NHS staff and new ways of working to meet patients' needs.

As can be seen from this historical overview, from 1942 when the Beveridge Report was published, the importance of partnerships between NHS organisations, social services, and the voluntary and private sectors has been recognised. However, up until 1997, when the White Paper, *The New NHS, Modern – Dependable* (Secretary of State for Health, 1997) was published the organisational structures and the ways in which the professions were working were not conducive to interprofessional working. Since 1997 this has been changing and new organisational structures and new ways of working have been evolving. Importantly, the new ways of working have meant that interprofessional working is no longer optional, it is mandatory.

As stated at the beginning of this historical overview, only the key health- and social-care policies related to interprofessional working have been discussed in this section. This section has not included those health- and social-care policies related to specific services, for example children's services and mental health services. For these two services, there have been many health- and social-care policies and legislation that have shaped the partnership approach taken to the care provided for patients.

What are the 'drivers' of interprofessional working?

Changes in professional practice do not occur in isolation, they are always located in a social, economic and political context. It is important to consider why we have interprofessional working and who benefits. In the past, while different professionals have worked alongside one another, caring for an individual patient, they were not seen as part of a team, and teamwork was, therefore, not evident.

Over recent years the requirement for health- and social-care professionals to work interprofessionally has become ever more evident, as the context within which health and social care is delivered has changed. The drivers for interprofessional working include:

1. The changing health- and social-care environment.
2. New government policies and initiatives.
3. High-profile child-abuse cases.
4. Professional developments.
5. Technological developments.

1. Changing health- and social-care environments

Patients are now being empowered to make informed decisions about their wellbeing, health and social care. The development of patient empowerment has occurred through both greater access to information and through cultural changes.

Technological developments, such as internet access, have significantly increased the information available to patients. No longer are patients basing their decisions only on information provided by local health- and social-care providers, they also have access to information across the world. To meet these changing needs and the expectations of patients, there is a requirement for more sophisticated approaches to the delivery of care involving effective teamwork, with health- and social-care professionals crossing boundaries and working interprofessionally.

Demographic changes have also impacted on how health- and social care are delivered within the UK. An ageing population with complex health- and social-care needs means that there is likely to be an increase in demand for health- and social-care provision. This increase in demand will also require care to be delivered in less traditional methods, with more and more care delivered within the community setting. Thus, it is essential that the different professionals working within the community setting (primary health care setting) collaborate with each other to provide effective health- and social care to those requiring it.

2. Government policy and initiatives

Over the last 10 years, the Department of Health has published many White Papers which have set out proposals to encourage teamwork and interprofessional working both between and within health- and social-care provision.

This trend in policies and initiatives continues with more recent government proposals focusing on improving the health of the population as a whole, with the emphasis being on preventative care. Initiatives such as NHS Direct, Walk-in Centres, Health Action Zones, Health Improvement Programmes and Healthy Living Centres have been implemented as part of these proposals. If these initiatives are to be successful in providing innovative approaches to health- and social care in the community, it is crucial that there is effective collaboration between the NHS, local authorities, social services and the private and voluntary sector.

These initiatives illustrate that the government continues to vehemently encourage and believe that effective interprofessional working will result in the effective delivery of patient-centred approaches to health- and social care.

The previous section, 'Historical overview of interprofessional developments', provides more detail on the health- and social-care policies and legislation that have shaped interprofessional working in the UK.

3. Child-abuse cases

The tragic deaths of young people as a result of abuse are all too frequently hitting the national headlines. In the UK, at least one child dies every week as a result of abuse. Many of these deaths never hit the national headlines, but they are no less tragic than those cases which do. Many other children suffer humiliating, dehumanising and degrading experiences from people on whom they are totally dependant, their main carers (Charles and Hendry, 2000).

One of the earliest reported deaths was that of Dennis O'Neill (Monckton Report, 1948, cited in Cretney, 1998) who died at the hands of his foster father. This was almost 60 years ago and yet the tragic deaths have continued to occur, one of the most recent being Victoria Climbié (Secretary of State for Health, 2003) who died at the hands of her aunt and her aunt's partner. Other tragic deaths include Maria Colwell, 1973; Jasmine Beckford, 1984; children undergoing heart surgery at Bristol Royal Infirmary, 1984–1995; Kimberley Carlie, 1986; Doreen Mason, 1987; Leanne White, 1992; Riki Neave, 1994; Chelsea Brown, 1999; Lauren Wright, 2000; and Ainlee Labonte, 2002.

Following the death of Dennis O'Neill in 1945, a Home Office inquiry (The Monkton Report, 1948) identified a string of failures by the staff and agencies involved in the case. There was confusion between the two local authorities responsible for Dennis O'Neill's foster placement, conflicting reports by childcare staff on his wellbeing, staff shortages and miscommunications.

The key messages from this report were that there needed to be better collaboration across organisational boundaries and improved communication between professionals.

Almost 30 years after the report into the death of Dennis O'Neill, the report into the death of Maria Colwell (Department of Health and Social Security, 1974, p. 86) concluded that the 'greatest and most obvious' failure of the system was 'the lack of, or effectiveness of communication and liaison'. This report also highlighted that the social worker involved in this case had a lack of knowledge and that training was, therefore, an issue. As can be seen, sadly, the same issues, lack of collaboration between agencies and lack of communication between professionals, which were present in 1948, were still present in 1974.

Another 30 years on from the death of Maria Colwell, the report into the death of Victoria Climbié (Secretary of State for Health, 2003) depressingly concluded by raising the same major issues. The Report, which concluded with 108 recommendations, highlighted a lack of collaborative working between agencies, a lack of effective sharing of information, and generally poor communication and lack of training of medical staff and in particular general practitioners (GPs).

In 2002, two years after the death of Victoria Climbié, Ainlee Labonte died. The report by Newham Area Child Protection Committee (2002) into her death had among its findings and conclusions the following:

- staff should receive better training to equip them to deal with violent families
- child-protection agencies need to improve the ways they work together to safeguard children at risk of abuse
- health, social services and the police failed to exchange information about the family, so no one gained a comprehensive picture of the danger Ainlee was in.

As can be seen, each new inquiry into a child's death over the last 60 years has resulted in a new but recurring set of recommendations. Sadly, it is apparent that the same issues exist today:

- lack of collaboration between agencies
- lack of effective communication
- lack of adequate training.

It is essential that the continuing deaths of children in such tragic circumstances are halted. While the issues relating to interprofessional working are not specific to child protection, there are two features in this area that make its achievement more difficult. Firstly, the development of the child-protection system has to a greater or lesser extent been influenced by the recommendations made by the public child-abuse enquiries. This has resulted in a series of initiatives coming from the Treasury, Department of Health and other government departments. These initiatives need to be coordinated into a set of policies by central government to provide an overarching coherent policy for the protection of vulnerable children. If this does not happen, the policies will be viewed as a series of quick fixes, which are unlikely to significantly improve interprofessional working. The second feature that makes achievement of interprofessional working more difficult is the wide range of agencies and professional groups involved.

However, underpinning the difficulties just described are fundamental organisational and structural problems, which need to be addressed in order to facilitate interprofessional working. When the Welfare State was created in the 1940s, health and social services were separated administratively at both central and local levels. This has meant that ever since the inception of the Welfare State, health and social services have had to make continual attempts to ensure their coordination. Over the years, health- and social-care policies have sought to encourage the coordinated planning of health and social services. Recently, however, this has gained momentum with the publication of documents such as *The New NHS, Modern – Dependable* (Secretary of State for Health, 1997); the creation of Care Trusts (Department of Health, 2000a); the introduction of 'flexibilities' (Department of Health, 1999a); *Modernising Social Services* (Department of Health, 1998a) and *Quality Strategy for Social Care* (Department of Health, 2000b). The significance of these health- and social-care policies and legislation for interprofessional working is discussed above in 'Historical overview of interprofessional developments'.

4. Professional developments

Health- and social-care provision has become increasingly complex to ensure that the needs of the patient continue to be met. Consequent to this growth in complexity, there has been an expansion in the knowledge and skills of those health and care professionals delivering the care. This expansion of knowledge has led to increased specialisation within the health- and social-care professions and new roles are being developed, for example clinical nurse specialists and consultant radiographers. As a result, teams with a greater skill-mix now deliver care to patients. If this team delivery approach is to be successful, effective interprofessional collaboration is essential.

The number of professionals available has also led to new specialist roles and subsequent new ways of working. For example, the current lack of availability of doctors means that if the traditional model of providing health- and social care is maintained, future expectations for the delivery of quality care are unlikely to be met. It is, therefore, more likely that the availability of professionals will shape future patterns of service delivery. Delivery will be provided in such a way that it ensures that the skills of all team members are used, by allowing them to contribute to their full potential.

Professional developments have impacted, and will continue to impact, on the nature of the delivery of care. These developments will inevitably mean that the traditional professional boundaries will be challenged as professionals cross the boundaries to deliver care to patients, using a team approach.

5. Technological developments

Although technological developments are not the drivers for interprofessional teamwork, they do have the potential to significantly enhance and influence interprofessional health- and social-care delivery. The use of information technology, for example mobile telephones, e-mail facilities, electronic patient records and video conferencing, will have a major impact on the development of interprofessional collaboration in primary health care. As members of primary health care teams are not usually geographically close to one another, advances in information technology will mean that information can be transferred more easily between members of the health care team. This will provide better opportunities for consultation between primary health care professionals, reduce professional isolation and should ultimately result in enhanced patient care.

Advances in telecommunications and information technology will inevitably have an important role to play in developing and sustaining interprofessional working.

Initiatives encouraging interprofessional working

In this section, we will discuss two examples of specific initiatives from the health- and social care sectors to explore the impact that health- and social-care policies and legislation have had on interprofessional working within the practice environment. The two initiatives selected are:

1. Health Action Zones.
2. Stroke.

1. Health Action Zones (HAZs)

HAZs were one of the initiatives for joint working that followed from the publication of the White Paper, *The New NHS, Modern – Dependable* (Department of Health, 1997). The purpose of a HAZ was to act as a catalyst to bring together in a working partnership all those contributing to the health of their local population, for example health organisations, local authorities, community groups, voluntary and private sectors, to implement locally agreed strategies for health.

HAZs were established in England in 1998 and 1999 and in total 26 HAZs were set up as seven-year pilot projects. All 26 HAZs shared common problems of social and economic deprivation, social exclusion and evidence of significant inequalities in health. Examples of HAZs include Luton and Bradford, which we will now look at briefly.

Luton

In Luton one of the priorities of the HAZ was addressing the health needs of Asian women, with a focus on increasing the uptake of cervical screening and developing a community-based colcoscopy service with a female consultant. There were five strategic working groups: health and social care; community capacity building; healthy environments; structural inequalities; and evaluation. Membership of these five working groups was drawn from the NHS, local government, the voluntary sector, academic and private organisations. In this HAZ, interprofessional collaboration produced joint guidelines for approaches to community development and joint working and training for the Borough Council and NHS staff involved in community development in the most deprived communities (Chirico *et al.*, 1998, cited in Amery, 2000).

Bradford

In Bradford, the objectives of the HAZ included a reduction in the incidence of cancer, diabetes, mental health problems, drug misuse and accidents. A particular focus was on diabetes, rehabilitation, improving the health of ethnic minorities and improving services in the inner city. Part of this initiative involved setting up a new community-based diabetes service, and also a partnership between the health authority, general practice, and community and acute trusts to deliver integrated preventative, specialist and primary care to a very needy population (Department of Health, 1999c).

As can be seen, the HAZs were created to initiate new ways of working, new partnerships, new financial arrangements and new structures within the health- and social-care sectors. To help the HAZs deliver new ways of working, targeted money was made available and a wide range of freedoms were introduced to enable them to operate more flexibly. These included:

- **New budgetary freedoms**. These included the ability to pool budgets between agencies, and freedom to move funds between budget headings, including capital and revenue budgets. It was also now permissable to move savings from one agency to another.

- **Joint planning**. This included opportunities to harmonise planning between local authority and NHS planning cycles, and freedom to develop common monitoring mechanisms across government initiatives.

Following completion of the seven-year pilot projects, the HAZs were incorporated into the developments of primary care trusts. A national evaluation of the action by HAZs to tackle inequalities of health was undertaken by Benzeval (2003). So, how successful were HAZs in breaking through organisational boundaries to tackle inequalities in health? Unfortunately, HAZs considered that their direct impact on health inequalities was minimal due to the short timeframe and limited resources. However, HAZs did include in their achievements the following:

- a broadened understanding of the determinants of health and a sense of ownership from a range of partners

- that they had helped develop partnership structures and collaborative working
- that they had helped develop more systematic planning processes.

This interprofessional initiative demonstrates that given the resources and the organisation and financial freedoms to work flexibly, new ways of working and new partnerships can be forged that have a positive impact on the quality of services provided to local communities.

2. Stroke

Stroke is the third most common cause of death in the UK and a major cause of disability in the population. Approximately 110 000 strokes occur in England each year and around half of all stroke survivors are left dependant on others for everyday activities. After-care is crucial to the patients' ability to recover and subsequent quality of life (National Audit Office, 2005).

The *National Service Framework for Older People* (Department of Health, 2001a) sets out eight national standards and service models of care regarding health- and social-care services for older people. The standards cover all older people whether they live at home, are in residential care or are being looked after in hospital.

The NSFs were developed following the publication of the White Paper, *A First Class Service: Quality in the New NHS* (Department of Health, 1998b). This White Paper set out plans to create a modern service that would deliver high-quality services for everyone through the setting and maintaining of national standards. The National Clinical Institute of Excellence was also developed following publication of this White Paper.

The NSF is a 10-year programme of improvement and will be implemented through a partnership between local health- and social-care providers. National programmes will underpin the local partnership activities. Progress will be monitored through a series of milestones and performance measures.

The NSF for older people was developed in partnership with older people and their carers, health- and social-care professionals, NHS and social services managers and partner agencies. Interprofessional collaboration with key stakeholders at this early stage is crucial. Involvement in the NSF development from its inception will mean that the key stakeholders will take ownership and have the necessary drive and ambition to see that the NSF is successfully implemented. As the key stakeholders are working collaboratively, they are also providing a role model for the health- and social-care professionals providing services at a local level.

Standard five of the NSF for older people refers to stroke. The aim of this standard is to reduce the incidence of stroke in the population and to ensure that those who have a stroke have prompt access to integrated stroke-care services. The Standard is as follows:

- the NHS will take action to prevent strokes, working in partnership with other agencies where appropriate
- people who are thought to have had a stroke have access to diagnostic services, are treated appropriately by a specialist stroke service and subsequently their carers participate in a multidisciplinary programme of secondary prevention and rehabilitation.

We can clearly see that to achieve this standard, effective interprofessional working is not just desirable but essential.

There are three strands to an integrated stroke service:

- stroke prevention for those at risk of a first or further stroke
- specialist stroke services providing acute care and rehabilitation
- long-term support for stroke patients and their carers.

In this section, we will primarily focus on strands two and three of the integrated stroke service, discussing the interprofessional approach taken to stroke care. Strand two refers to the development of specialist stroke services. The NSF Standard five requires that all general hospitals that care for people who have had a stroke must have a specialist stroke service. This is because it is recognised that the outcomes for stroke patients are better when they are cared for by a specialist stroke team, within a dedicated acute and rehabilitation stroke unit. The key components of the specialist stroke service include:

- a specialist stroke team
- an acute stroke unit
- a stroke rehabilitation unit.

The specialist stroke team is a large interprofessional team and its membership typically includes:

- Stroke physician
- Stroke nurse consultant
- Occupational therapists
- Nursing staff
- Pharmacists
- Stroke-care coordinator
- Clinical psychologist
- Physiotherapist
- Social worker
- Speech and language therapist
- Community neuro-rehabilitation team.

The specialist stroke-care team working within a specialist acute and rehabilitation stroke unit will offer an integrated stroke service, as follows:

○━ィ Keywords

Multidisciplinary team (MDT)

A group of people of different professions who meet on a regular basis to discuss individual patients. Each different professional contributes independently to the diagnostic treatment or care decisions regarding each patient case

- The service will provide patient-focused care
- It will be ensured that the specialist stroke team will assess each patient as soon as they are admitted to hospital with a stroke
- The team will hold **multidisciplinary team (MDT)** meetings each week. At the MDT meeting, each patient will be discussed in detail, which gives all the members of the team an opportunity to understand the current progress in all aspects of their patients' care. The MDT meeting also enables the future care and treatment of patients to be discussed, planned and agreed (see Chapter 5 for further detail on MDT meetings.)
- Carers and family members will be encouraged to participate in care right from the start. This enables more effective communication with the family and carers and facilitates the setting of realistic goals.

Education is a key factor in all aspects of stroke-care provision. The interprofessional environment within which stroke care is offered provides an ideal interprofessional learning opportunity. In some specialist stroke units, monthly interprofessional education symposiums or journal clubs have been established. The specialist stroke teams are also responsible for developing and providing education programmes both within the hospital and in the community setting for members of the general public. Programmes include, for example, learning about stroke and stroke prevention. Often these programmes will be supplemented by written information.

When working within an interprofessional team such as the specialist stroke team, there is also the opportunity to develop a joint staff-training programme.

As we can see, the specialist stroke team is an excellent example of an interprofessional team working and learning together to provide a quality service to stroke patients and their family and carers. The specialist stroke team does not, however, work in isolation and once the patient leaves the rehabilitation stroke unit, their care continues in the community. The rehabilitation services offered in the community are wide and varied and include:

- Day-care social services
- Dietetics
- Musculoskeletal physiotherapy
- Speech and language therapy
- District nursing service
- Wheelchair services
- Social-care occupational therapy services
- Leisure centre.

The voluntary sector is an important part of the interprofessional team caring for patients who have suffered a stroke and their family and carers. The Stroke Association, for example, is a national charity covering England and Wales that offers a wide range of services to those affected by stroke, including a Family Support Service, Dysphasia Support Service and a Prevention Service. The Stroke Association also works closely with statutory health and social services organisations to reduce the impact of stroke. For example, the Stroke Association produces booklets and a series of resource packs for health- and social-care professionals working with those affected by stroke (The Stroke Association, 2006).

Other voluntary associations that work with those affected by stroke include:

- **Different Strokes**. This is run by and for younger people who have had strokes
- **Connect – the Communication Disability Network**. This organisation works with people living with stroke and **aphasia**
- **Speakability**. This is a national charity that supports people living with aphasia and their carers.

○━┓ Keywords

Aphasia
Is the loss of the ability to use and understand language; it can be speaking, writing or listening. It is usually caused by stroke, brain disease or injury

Evidence base

Go to the following websites and read about the services that these organisations provide for those affected by stroke:

- The Stroke Association www.stroke.org.uk
- Different Strokes www.differentstrokes.co.uk
- Connect – the Communication Disability Network www.ukconnect.org
- Speakability www.speakability.org.uk.

This discussion has illustrated the impact that health- and social-care policies have had on the care provided to those people who have suffered a stroke and their family and carers. The development of an integrated stroke service has meant that a wide range of health- and social-care professionals are now committed to interprofessional working and learning and are collaborating effectively to provide a patient-focused service.

Stroke was also one of the priorities set out in the White Paper *Saving lives: Our Healthier Nation* (Department of Health, 1999d). One of the targets was to reduce the death rate from coronary disease, stroke and related diseases in people under 75 years by at least two-fifths by 2010, saving up to 200,000 lives. Stroke is also referred to in the *National Service Framework for Coronary Heart Disease* (Department of Health, 2001c) and the *National Service Framework for Long-term Conditions* (Department of Health, 2005).

RRRRRRapid recap

Check your progress so far by working through each of the following questions.

1. What are the five drivers for interprofessional working?
2. What three factors are still inhibiting successful interprofessional working?
3. What was the purpose of developing Health Action Zones?
4. What three main Department of Health policies have impacted on the delivery of stoke services in the UK?

If you have difficulty with more than one of the questions, read through the section again to refresh your understanding before moving on.

References

Amery, J. (2000) Interprofessional Working in Health Action Zones: How Can This be Fostered. *Journal of Interprofessional Care*, **14**(1): 27–30.

Benzeval, M. (2003) *The Final Report of the Tackling Inequalities in Health Module: The National Evaluation of Health Action Zones. A Report to the Department of Health.* Queen Mary College, University of London, London. Available from: www.geog.qmul.ac.uk/health/publications/index.html.

Charles, M. and Hendry, E. (2000) *Training Together to Safeguard Children: Guidance on Interagency Training.* NSPCC, London.

Cretney, S. (1998) *Law, Law Reform and the Family.* Clarendon Press, Gloucestershire.

Department of Health (1989a) *Working for Patients.* Department of Health, London.

Department of Health (1989b) *Caring for People: Community Care in the Next Decade and Beyond.* Department of Health, London.

Department of Health (1998a) *Modernising Social Services: Promoting Independence, Improving Protection, Raising Standards.* Department of Health, London. Available from: www.dh.gov.uk/publications.

Department of Health (1998b) *A First Class Service: Quality in the NHS.* Department of Health, London.

Department of Health (1999a) *Health Act 1999 – Modern Partnerships for People.* Department of Health, London.

Department of Health (1999b) *Agenda for Change: Modernising the NHS Pay System.* Department of Health, London.

Department of Health (1999c) *Health Action Zones in 78 Million Pound Trailblazing of Money for Modernisation.* Press Release: Reference number 1999/0034. Available from: www.dh.gov.uk/PublicationsAndStatistics/PressReleases/PressReleasesNotices/fs/en?CONTENT_ID=4025111&chk=%2BBY0kZ.htm.

Department of Health (1999d) *Saving Lives: Our Healthier Nation.* Department of Health, London.

Department of Health (2000a) *The NHS Plan: a plan for investment, a plan for reform.* Department of Health, London. Available from: www.dh.gov.uk/publications.

Department of Health (2000b) *A Quality Strategy for Social Care.* Department of Health, London. Available from: www.dh.gov.uk/publications.

Department of Health (2001a) *National Service Framework for Older People*. Department of Health, London. Available from: www.dh.gov.uk/publications.

Department of Health (2001b) *Health- and Social-Care Act 2001*. Department of Health, London.

Department of Health (2001c) *National Service Framework for Coronary Heart Disease*. Department of Health, London. Available from: www.dh.gov.uk/publications.

Department of Health (2003) *The NHS Knowledge and Skills Framework (KSF) and the Development Review Guidance – Working Draft (March 2003)*. Department of Health, London.

Department of Health (2004a) *National Service Framework for Children, Young People and Maternity Services*. Department of Health, London. Available from: www.dh.gov.uk/publications.

Department of Health (2004b) *The NHS Improvement Plan: Putting People at the Heart of Public Services*. Department of Health, London. Available from: www.dh.gov.uk/publications.

Department of Health (2005) *National Service Framework for Long-term (Neurological) Conditions*. Department of Health, London. Available from: www.dh.gov.uk/publications.

Department of Health and Social Security (1990) *National Health Service & Community Care Act*. HMSO, London.

Department of Health and Social Security (1974) *Report of the Committee of Enquiry into the Care and Supervision Provided in Relation to Maria Colwell*. HMSO, London.

Headrick, L.A., Wilcock, M. and Batalden, B. (1998) Interprofessional Working and Continuing Medical Education. *BMJ*, **316**: 771–774.

Hugman, R. (1995) Contested Territory and Community Services: Interprofessional Boundaries in Health- and social-care. In *Interprofessional Relations in Health Care* (eds. Soothill, K., Mackay, L. and Webb, C. Edward Arnold, London.

Lymbery, M. (1998) Social Work in General Practice: Dilemmas and Solutions. *Journal of Interprofessional Care*, **12**(2): 199–208.

National Audit Office (1999) *Modernising Government White Paper*. HMSO, London.

National Audit Office (2005) *Reducing Brain Damage: Faster Access to Better Stroke Care*. National Audit Office, London. Available from: www.nao.org.uk/pn/05–06/0506452.htm.

Newham Area Child Protection Committee (2002) *Ainlee Born: 24.06.1999 : Died: 07.01.2002 Chapter 8 Review*. Newham Area Child Protection Committee, Newham. Available from: www.newham.gov.uk/NR/rdonlyres/3494306C-1D26-4D28-B0CD-5020B93CAD41/0/AinleeLabonte.pdf.

Secretary of State for Health (1997) *The New NHS, Modern – Dependable*. The Stationery Office, London. Available from: www.dh.gov.uk/publications.

Secretary of State for Health (2003) *The Victoria Climbié Inquiry*. The Stationery Office, London.

The Stroke Association (2006) A variety of books and resource packs available from: www.stroke.org.uk.

World Health Organization (1978) *Alma Ata 1978 Primary Care*. World Health Organization, Geneva.

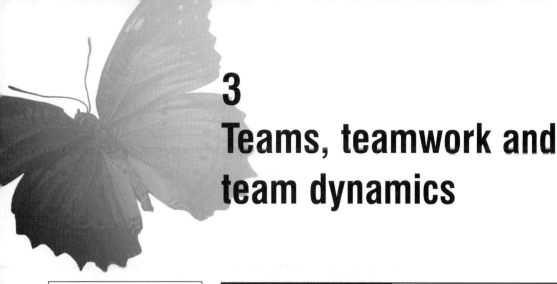

3 Teams, teamwork and team dynamics

Learning outcomes

By the end of this chapter you should be able to:

★ Describe and define the different types of team

★ Identify what helps and hinders effective teamwork

★ Discuss the potential benefits of working in a team

★ Understand the key criteria for evaluating the effectiveness of teams.

Teams and teamwork

The need for teams and effective teamwork within and between the health- and social-care sectors is crucial to improving the productivity of health- and social-care professionals and the quality of care that they provide.

The concept of teams and teamwork features prominently within the literature on interprofessional working. The definition of a team and teamwork are often taken for granted, but these terms mean different things to different people. It is therefore important when you are developing a team to find out what the other team members' views of what a team and teamwork are and how they value team working.

What is a team?

Within the literature relating to teams and teamwork there are many differing definitions of a team. Two examples of attempts to define a team are given below:

> A team is a group of people who make different contributions towards the achievement of a common goal.
>
> Pritchard and Pritchard (1994, p. 13)

> A team is a small number of people with complementary skills who are committed to a common purpose, performance goals, and approach for which they hold themselves mutually accountable.
>
> Katzenbach and Smith (1993, p. 45)

If these two definitions along with the many others found within the literature are examined, the essential characteristics of a team emerge. Let us now consider what these 'essential' features of a team are. A team is a group of people who:

• share a common purpose and common goals

• have a clear understanding of each other's roles and abilities

• are task oriented and have different, but complementary skills

- have a shared knowledge, skills and resource base, and collective responsibility for the outcome of their decisions.

When considering an interprofessional team one further characteristic needs to be added to the above list of 'essential' characteristics:

- composed of persons from differing professions and/or organisations who work together to benefit the patient and their significant others.

What is teamwork?

The literature relating to teamwork reveals many definitions of teamwork. Two examples are given below:

> Co-ordinated action carried out by two or more individuals jointly, concurrently or sequentially. It implies common agreed goals, clear awareness of, and respect for others' roles and functions. On the part of each member of the team, adequate human and material resources, supportive co-operative relationships and mutual trust, effective leadership, open, honest and sensitive communications, and provision for evaluations.
>
> Kekki (1990)

> Teamwork is the way people work together cooperatively and effectively.
>
> Manion *et al.* (1996)

If we review the definitions of teamwork, recurrent themes can be identified. These can provide us with the essential characteristics of teamwork. Teamwork involves:

- having a common purpose and common objectives
- delegation and empowerment
- different professional contributions
- having systems in place to facilitate effective communication
- coordination, cooperation and joint thinking
- focusing on the patient to provide the best means of serving patient/client interests
- allowing team members to carry out the team's work and to manage itself as an independent group of people.

How does a team develop?

When a team is developing it will usually go through a series of stages before becoming really effective. It is useful to know the stages in team development, so that when your team appears to be going nowhere or members of the team are constantly arguing, you understand that this is normal! Understanding the stages will enable you to work towards moving the team on to the next stage.

Five stages of team development have been identified. They are forming, storming, norming, performing and adjourning (Tuckman and Jenson, 1977).

Forming

When a team is forming, the team members spend time getting to know each other and individual team members avoid controversy, due to wanting to be accepted by the team. Team members may feel anxious because they do not know how the group will work or what exactly will be required of them.

During this stage the team members define the common objectives of the team and discussion centres on how the team are going to tackle achieving the agreed objective.

For the team to move from this stage to the next, team members must give up the comfort of safe, non-threatening topics and risk the possibility of conflict.

Storming

As the name of this stage suggests, this is the time when things within the team may get stormy. Team members test each other, they question values and behaviours, the worth and feasibility of the common objectives may be challenged, as well as who is responsible for what. The guidance and direction of the leader may also be challenged. As a result of the discomfort generated by the conflict some members may withdraw and remain completely silent, while others may attempt to dominate.

If storming is not allowed to happen the team may never perform effectively. Storming is a healthy process in which the team evolves with a common set of values, believes and objectives.

In order to move from this stage to the next, team members must move from testing each other and conflict to 'listening to each other and problem solving'. Some teams never get beyond the storming stage in their development and may disintegrate because conflict between the team members cannot be resolved.

Norming

During this stage the team starts to function harmoniously and individuals in the team value the differences that other members bring to the team. Team members are more willing to change their preconceived ideas or opinions on the basis of facts presented to them by other team members and members actively ask questions of one another.

Creativity is high during this stage with team members sharing feelings and ideas, asking and giving feedback to one another and exploring activities related to the common objectives of the team. Cooperation and collaboration replace the conflict and mistrust felt by the team members during the stormy stage of development.

Some teams do not go beyond the norming stage of development.

Performing

When a team successfully reaches the performing stage, it will be working effectively and efficiently together to meet the team's common objectives. The team is now at its most productive, with the team and individual team members learning and developing together.

The performing stage can lead into a return to the forming stage if the team membership changes or to the final stage of development, adjourning.

Adjourning

This stage marks the end of the working life of the team, with the team successfully reaching its common objectives and its work completed. The dismantling of a team can create a minor crisis for individual team members with team members feeling sad, nostalgic and 'mourning' the end of a team. The most effective interventions during the adjourning stage are those that help the team to tie up loose ends.

Although all teams pass through these five stages during their development, all teams develop at their own pace and in their own unique way. These stages may be longer or shorter for each team, or for individual members of the team. The formation of teams also differs; some teams can be represented as a spiral, while other teams form with sudden movements forward and then have periods of no change.

Health- and social-care teams are complex and dynamic and while the professional groups that make up the team normally remain fairly static, the individuals representing each profession may change on a more frequent basis. As a result, team development is not a straightforward linear process and the addition of new team members may cause the team to go back to the forming stage. Team development is likely to be 'stop-start' rather than a smooth development. It is important to recognise that new team members will not always result in the team going back to the forming stage; the team may stay at the same stage or may go back to the storming or norming stage of development dependant on the stage of team development reached before the new member joins the team. New team members will, however, always affect the dynamics of the team that they are joining. The impact of a new member on the team is not necessarily negative of course, and may be beneficial to the continuing development of the team.

Reflective activity

Think of a team that you have recently been involved with and use the questions below to help you reflect on your team's development.

1 Forming

- What were the common objectives of the team?
- Did you all share the same expectations of the common objectives?
- Did you all have the same attitude to working in the team?
- Did you feel any anxiety on joining the team?

2 Storming

- Was there any conflict in the team?
- Did you all agree on how to tackle the common objectives?
- Was the authority of the team leader challenged?
- Did any team members withdraw from the team?

3 Norming

- Were the team members willing to change their preconceived ideas/opinions?
- Did you feel able to ask for and give constructive feedback to other team members?
- Did you cooperate with each other?
- Did you work out how to proceed?

4 Performing

- Did you work effectively and efficiently?
- Did the team focus on achieving the common objectives?
- Did you experience a sense of achievement?

5 Adjourning

- Did the team stop abruptly and you all go your own separate ways or did you successfully achieve the common objectives and go off together and socialise?
- Did you talk about the team and your experience of it?
- What sort of issues did you discuss or think about after the team dismantled?

What types of people are in teams?

When considering interprofessional teams it is important to understand what an individual brings to a team. This will enable you to reflect on your preferred team role, the roles that other team members may take on and the impact that these roles have on both your behaviour towards others and the behaviour of others towards you.

Benne and Skeats (1948, cited in Payne, 2000) were some of the earliest writers to describe team roles. They divided team roles into three types:

- those roles involving task functions
- those roles involving maintenance functions
- those roles involving the individual.

Roles involving task functions

These roles emphasise getting the job done and relate to the common objectives of the team.

Roles involving team maintenance

These roles emphasise keeping the team working together in harmony, dealing with conflict and issues of team maintenance.

Table 3.1 Roles involving task functions

Initiator	Proposes new ideas, new tasks, new methods
Information-giver	Gives or volunteers to find out information
Clarifier	Takes individual contributions and clarifies; encourages people to be specific
Elaborator	Expands on existing suggestions
Coordinator	Helps pull ideas and themes together
Evaluator	Critically evaluates ideas, proposals and plans
Summariser	Summarises what has been achieved
Questioner	Asks fundamental questions about the common objectives and challenges assumptions

Table 3.2 Roles involving team maintenance

Encourager	Offers praise and agreement with other members; warm and understanding
Harmoniser	Mediates conflict and disagreements that occur
Compromiser	Seeks a compromise that all parties can accept
Standard setter	States or applies team standards
Gate keeper	Encourages others to participate; limits lengthy contributions
Team observer – commentator	Feeds back interpretations of team process
Follower	Accepts direction of group process

Roles involving the individual

These roles relate to the personality of the individual.

Table 3.3 Roles involving the individual

Aggressor	Attacks or criticises; deflates others' status
Blocker	Negative; disagrees without reason
Dominator	Exerts authority; interrupts
Self confessor	Expresses irrelevant personal feelings to receive attention
Help seeker	Seeks sympathy through expressing insecurity or confusion
Playboy	Cynical; lack of involvement
Special-interest pleader	Masks own biases through pleading on behalf of others
Recognition seeker	Seeks attention; seeks important roles

Since Benne and Skeats (1948, cited in Payne, 2000) identified the different types of roles found within a team, numerous teamwork writers have adapted their typology. However, the three roles related to task, team maintenance and the individual have remained.

Although Benne and Skeats' (1948, cited in Payne 2000) work has been significant, it is important when using these team roles to remember the following:

- the role descriptors describe patterns of behaviour within a team and not necessarily particular people or personality types
- an individual can adopt different roles at different times and in different situations, depending on the skills of the other team members
- team members may take on helpful and unhelpful roles at the same time.

It was not until the early 1980s that a completely new approach was taken to defining team roles. This work was undertaken by Dr Meredith Belbin, whose research examined the roles taken within the work tasks that a team undertake. Belbin's (1981) work originated from a management training exercise, in which over 200 simulated teams were set up to carry out tasks in groups. Following many years of research, nine roles were identified, which were considered necessary if a team was to be successful. These roles are set out in Table 3.4.

Belbin (1981) clustered these nine team-role types into three groups:

1. **Action-oriented roles**: Shaper, Implementer and Completer-finisher
2. **People-oriented roles**: Coordinator, Teamworker and Resource-Investigator
3. **Cerebral roles**: Plant, Monitor Evaluator and Specialist.

Table 3.4 Belbin's Team Roles

Role	Personality traits	Contributions	Possible weaknesses
Implementer	Methodical Practical Conscientious Reliable	Turns ideas into practical actions	Inflexible Conservative Lacks imagination Does not inspire or motivate others
Shaper	Challenging Dynamic Thrives on pressure Opportunistic	Driving force Makes things happen Galvanises team	Impatient Offends people's feelings Argues or disagrees
Plant	Creative Clever Loner Radical Original Unorthodox	Produces imaginative ideas Solves difficult problems	Disregards practical details Unrealistic Can be isolated or become a scapegoat
Resource-investigator	Extrovert Relaxed Sociable Communicative Enthusiastic	Explores opportunities Develops contacts Good negotiator	Over-optimistic Tendency to lose interest once initial enthusiasm has passed
Monitor evaluator	Judicious Analytical Prudent Unemotional Dispassionate	Judges accurately Sees all options Helps the team avoid mistakes	May appear dry, boring, over-critical Lacks ability to inspire and motivate others
Teamworker	Cooperative Diplomatic Sympathetic Sociable Avoids conflict	Promotes harmony and team spirit Averts disputes Puts team before self	Indecisive in moments of crisis Reluctant to do things that might hurt others
Completer-finisher	Painstaking Anxious Conscientious Ordering	Dots the 'i's' and crosses the 't's' Gives attention to detail Delivers on time	Inclined to worry unduly Has difficulty letting go or delegating work Over-perfectionist
Coordinator	Mature Confident Good chairperson	Committed to team goals and objectives Promotes decision-making Delegates well	Can be seen as manipulative Offloads personal work
Specialist	Single-minded Self-starting Dedicated Committed	Provides knowledge and skills which are in rare supply	Contributes only on a narrow front Dwells on technicalities Lacks interest in other people's subjects

As with Benne and Skeat's work (1948, cited in Payne, 2000), Belbin's team role types should be used with caution. It is important to remember when a new team is developing that almost always people have a mix of roles and will have dominant and sub-dominant roles. Belbin's work provides a useful introduction to the idea of team roles, but its practical use in team building is limited.

More recent approaches to identifying team roles have focused on skills rather than personality types. For example, Margerison and McCann (1995) identified eight role preferences following discussions with successful teams. Table 3.5 identifies these role preferences.

Table 3.5 Role preferences focusing on skills

Creator–innovators	Independent people who come up with ideas
Explorer–promoters	Sociable people who bring ideas, contacts and resources
Assessor–developers	Practical people who get ideas to work and test them against practical requirements
Thruster–organisers	Motivators who organise people and systems
Concluder–producers	Consistent people who maintain quality standards
Controller–inspectors	Careful people who check and evaluate work
Upholder–maintainers	Stable people who support others
Reporter–advisers	Patient people who are good at collecting and presenting information

Although recent analyses of team roles claim to focus on skills and not on personalities, it is apparent that many of the descriptors for team role types do have elements of personality styles within them. For example, in Table 3.5, explorer–promoters are described as 'sociable' people while upholder–maintainers are described as 'stable' people.

If we look back at the team role types described in this section, Benne and Skeats (1948, cited in Payne, 2000), Belbin (1981) and Margerison and McCann (1995), what is evident is that they bear remarkable similarities to each other. This would suggest that the research undertaken into team roles over the last 60 years has resulted in well-established categorisations of personalities from work and also that there is a consistent pattern of role division in the workplace.

Despite the criticisms levied at team role descriptors, this type of analysis can be useful to both the individual team member and the team. For the individual, being aware of their team role type provides an opportunity for professional development facilitating growth of the individual by learning new and additional roles to take up within the team. For the team, role analysis helps team members to see beyond defining other team members merely by their profession or job role. It enables team members to identify and appreciate the wider contributions that they and other team members make to the team.

Refle**Reflective activity**

Think about two teams that you have been a member of in the last three months. One team should be an interprofessional work team and the other a team from your personal life. For each team consider the following points.

● List the dominant and sub-dominant team roles that you took up.

● Did you take up different dominant and sub-dominant team roles in each team?

● If so, why do you think that this happened?

● Using Belbin's model, identify the dominant team role that individual team members took up.

● Did each team have the nine team roles identified by Belbin? If so, was the team successful?

If your team had team roles missing, what impact did this have on the success of your teams?

How are teams described?

It is important that the distinctions between different types of team are understood, so that we know what type of team we are in and how we can develop the team to ensure that the team continues to meet the needs of specific patient groups and the requirements of the health- and social-care services.

Two models for categorising different types of team will be described.

Katzenbach and Smith's model

Katzenbach and Smith (1993) developed a model that differentiates between different types of team and different levels of performance according to a performance curve. This model is shown in Figure 3.1.

As Figure 3.1 illustrates, this model has five different types of team.

Working group

This type of group shares information and best practices to make decisions to help each individual to function within their own area of responsibility. There is little shared responsibility.

Pseudo-team

A pseudo-team is one where the team members have no interest in agreeing a common goal for the team, but they still call themselves a team. In a pseudo-team, the sum of the whole is less than the potential of the individual parts. Pseudo-teams are often less effective than

Figure 3.1 Different types of team and their different levels of performance

Reprinted by permission of Harvard Business School Press. From *The Wisdom of Teams: Creating The High Performance Organization* by J. R. Katzenbach and D. K. Smith. Boston, MA. Copyright © 1993 by the Harvard Business School Publishing Corporation; all rights reserved.

working groups because they have nothing concrete to do as a team that will contribute to the service/organisation.

Potential team

In a potential team the team members can see the need to improve performance. However, the team members require greater clarity about the purpose and goals of the team and need to work out a common approach.

The steepest performance gain comes between a potential and a real team.

Real team

A real team is a small number of people with different but complementary skills, who are committed to a common purpose and common goals and who take collective responsibility for the outcome of their decisions.

High-performance team

This type of team has all the characteristics of a real team but in addition it has team members who are committed to one another's personal growth and success.

Øvretveit's (1997) model

Øvretveit's (1997) model for describing a team is particularly helpful because it relates specifically to interprofessional working in the health- and social-care sectors. This model puts forward four ways in which a team can be defined.

Membership

It is important to agree who is in the team and who is not in the team and why. Øvretveit (1997) distinguishes between 'core' and 'associate' membership, the former usually referring to full-time membership and the latter referring to part-time membership.

The mix of different professions in a team and how many of each is in the team is another important consideration. If the mix of professions and the number of professionals is right then the skills of the team should match the individual needs of the patient.

The experience, status and seniority of the team membership must also be recognised to ensure that the experience that individuals bring to the team is valued. This is an important aspect of team membership, as this knowledge will help in matching team members with patients and will also help in determining individual team members' needs for professional development.

Team process

A patient passes through a number of stages on their journey to and through a team. At each stage, decisions about the patient's care are made. The way in which the team makes these decisions reflects the type of team process that the team has adopted, and hence the patient pathway that the patient will follow. Øvretveit (1997) identifies six common types of team process: parallel pathway team; allocation team; reception-and-allocation team; reception-assessment-allocation-team; reception-assessment-allocation-review team; and hybrid-parallel-pathway team. Although the way in which a team makes decisions is different for each pathway, all the patients pass through the same stages in their care pathway:

Referral → Assessment → Care Plan → Review → Case closed

Management structure

The management structure of a team, that is, how the team is led and how the practitioners within that team are managed, is another way in which an interprofessional team can be described. Øvretveit (1997) identifies five team management structures.

Profession-managed

In this type of management structure, the members from each profession are separately managed by a manager from their own profession. In an interprofessional team, this may mean that members of the team are managed by separate agencies as well as separate departments. In a primary health care team for example, team members may have managers from social services (if they are social workers), education (if they are special needs teachers) and from the health services (if they are nurses, physiotherapists or community midwives).

Single manager

In this case, team members from different professions are all managed by the same team manager (taken from one of the professions). In a single-manager structure, there may also be professional advisers to help the manager with professional issues.

Joint management

In this management structure, there is a team coordinator who organises the work of the team, but each practitioner also relates to a manager from their own profession on professional issues.

Team manager-contracted

The team manager has a budget to buy services from professionally managed services.

Hybrid management

As the name suggests this is a mixed management structure, with the team manager managing core staff, joint management responsibilities over other members of the team, and contracting in additional members to the team.

Integration

Another way to describe a team is by considering the extent to which the team members are integrated into the team. The greater the degree of integration, then the closer the working relationship between the different professions within the team will be.

Reflective activity

Think about an interprofessional team in which you are a member of the team. Using Katzenbach and Smith (1993) and Øvretveit's (1997) models consider the following points.

- What type of interprofessional team are you in?
- Would the team be more effective if it operated as a different type of team? If so, what type of team?
- How do you think you could develop your team to enhance the services it provides to patients?

Key points Top tips

The advantages of interprofessional teams and teamworking are:

- A more responsive and patient-centred service
- Avoids duplication of work and fragmentation of the service
- More effective and efficient use of staff, which leads to more satisfying roles and career pathways for health- and social-care professionals
- A more effective service provision through improved organisation and planning.

What does an interprofessional team look like?

There are many examples of interprofessional teams working within the health- and social-care sector. Two examples of interprofessional teams that have developed significantly in recent years are primary health care teams and palliative-care teams.

Primary health care teams

Primary health care has been defined by the World Health Organization declaration of Alma Ata (WHO, 1978) as:

> the first level contact of individuals, the family and the community with the national health system which brings health care as close as possible to where people live and work, and constitutes the first element of a continuing health process.

A primary health care team can, therefore, be described as a group of professionals delivering health services in the community at the first point of contact with the health service. Table 3.6 indicates those health- and social-care professionals typically considered to form part of a primary health care team.

As the table illustrates, a primary health care team is larger than the optimum team size of eight to 10 members. If, however, the structure of the primary health care team is examined, it can be seen that different types of team are operating. There are large network structures, which include both health- and social-care professionals. Within these networks, communication tends to be intermittent and team members will network with each other as and when the need arises. More formally structured teams exist, which are based around general medical practices. These teams will be smaller with 10 to 15 members and communication will be tighter than that which occurs within the networks, although as with networks, communication will be broad. Finally, small individual patient-centred teams exist, which tend to be task based and time limited. Communication within these teams is frequent, full, but narrower, as it is focused on specific patient issues (Royal Pharmaceutical Society of Great Britain and the British Medical Association, 2000).

This range of different team types means that individuals could be contributing as members of different teams at different times, or even at the same time (see Figure 3.2).

Table 3.6 Members of a primary health care team

● General practitioners	● Diabetic specialist nurse
● Practice managers	● Occupational health nurses
● Practice nurses	● Audiologists
● Nurse practitioners	● Paramedics
● Community nurses	● Macmillan nurses
● Community midwives	● Community matrons
● Health visitors	● Podiatry
● Allied health professionals	● Community pharmacist
● Social workers	● Stoma nurses
● Receptionists	● Falls prevention coordinator
● Administrative and clerical staff	● Dentists
● Counsellors	● Opticians
● Outside agencies e.g. Age Concern, Marie Curie, Crossroads, Private Home-Care Agencies	● School nurses

NB The list of professionals included in this table is by no means exhaustive as the professionals included in a primary health care team vary from region to region. The members are not listed in any specific order.

Reflective activity

Think about your local primary health care team and consider the following points from both a professional and patient viewpoint:

● Which members of your primary health care team have you come into contact with?

● What types of primary health care teams did/do you come into contact with?

● Draw a diagram(s) to illustrate the different types of team and the team members that you have come into contact with.

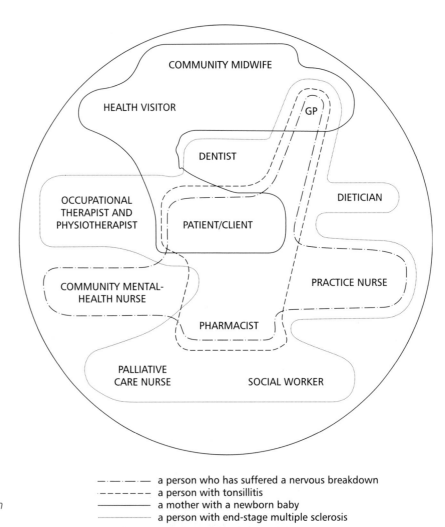

- — · — · — a person who has suffered a nervous breakdown
- — — — — a person with tonsillitis
- ———— a mother with a newborn baby
- ················ a person with end-stage multiple sclerosis

*Figure 3.2 How primary
health care teams might form
around specific patients*

Case study

Teams and effective communication

Chris is a community nurse who works in a rural county. She rarely meets with her colleagues within the primary health care team. Her main form of communication with other members of the team is via the telephone or, more frequently, through the patient's electronic record. Mrs Smith, a patient Chris sees on a daily basis to dress and clean her leg ulcer, also has a 'communication book'. Mrs Smith takes this communication book to all her appointments and this enables Chris to communicate with other health care professionals caring for Mrs Smith and for other health care professionals to communicate with Chris. Chris does feel very isolated and does not feel part of a team. She would like to discuss this with her team leader and the rest of the team.

1. What type of team do you think Chris is in?
2. How do you think Chris could improve her communication channels with the rest of her team?
3. What needs to happen to make Chris feel that she is part of her team?
4. Suggest a team-building exercise that would be useful for Chris's team.

Palliative-care teams

Palliative care is the active care of patients whose disease is not responsive to curative treatment. The aim of palliative care is to provide the best possible quality of life to patients and their carers. This is achieved through effective symptom control, encompassing the control of pain and other symptoms, as well as the psychological, social and spiritual aspects of the patient.

The aim of a palliative-care team is to provide quality care for patients requiring palliative care, in both the primary and secondary care settings. Table 3.7 illustrates the health- and social-care professionals that make up a typical palliative-care team and provides a brief description of the role of each professional.

As Table 3.7 illustrates, a palliative-care team, like a primary health care team is larger than the widely believed optimum size for a team to function effectively (eight to 10 people). It may be more appropriate to call both these teams an enterprise, that is, a palliative-care enterprise and a primary health care enterprise. The term 'enterprise' is used when a team has more than 40 members.

If the structure of the palliative-care team is considered, it can be seen that, as with the primary health care team, different types of team are operating. The focus of these different types of team, as with any health- or social-care team, is the patient and their significant others. Thus, the health- and social-care professionals that make up the palliative-care team caring for a patient will depend on the type and progress of the disease, as well as the social and psychological care that the patient requires at any one point of time. This means that while there will be a 'core' team caring for a patient's palliative-care needs, the team will expand as and when appropriate. For example, if a patient with terminal breast cancer develops painful bony metastases in their thoracic vertebrae, they may be offered radiotherapy to control the pain. At this point, the palliative-care team caring for this patient would expand to include, for example, an oncologist, therapeutic radiographers and a Macmillan radiographer. As this example illustrates, individual health- or social-care professionals will be members of different patient-centred care teams at the same time.

The primary health care team and palliative-care team are just two examples of interprofessional teams found in the health- and social-care sector. Both these examples demonstrate the complexity of interprofessional health- and social-care teams, providing some insight into the challenges that face professionals in working effectively as part of such a large, complex and changing team.

Table 3.7 Members of a typical palliative-care team

Place of care	Team	Role
Community	Primary health care team with the addition of specialist palliative-care involvement which may include: ● Specialist palliative-care nurse (often referred to as a Macmillan nurse)	● Advises and provides support to the patient and their family and other professionals
	● Hospice at home	● This may be a stand-alone team or attached to a hospice or palliative-care team ● Provides clinical care and support, often in symptom management of end-of-life issues
	● Specialist palliative-care physician	● Provides advice and assessment in complex symptom management ● May visit the patient at home or may see the patient as an outpatient
	● Marie Curie Nurses (Charitable Fund)	● Provide sitting and hands-on care for patients, as respite for main carer at end of life
Hospital	Secondary health care team with the addition of: ● Specialist palliative-care physician and an attached team	● Assesses and treats patients referred by other clinicians
	● Specialist palliative-care nurse (often referred to as a Macmillan nurse)	● Advise and provide support for the patient and their family and other professionals
	● Oncology nurses	● Provide advice and support to the patient and their family and other professionals on site-specific issues, for example breast, prostate or haematology problems
	● Complementary therapists	● Provide a range of therapies, massage, counselling
	● Lymphoedema specialist nurse	● Provides care and treatment for patients with lymphoedema
Hospice or hospice-at-home team	This is usually a charitable institution with varying amounts of money given by the local NHS Trusts. The hospice team will include: ● Registered nurses ● Doctors ● Pharmacist ● Counsellor ● Occupational therapist ● Physiotherapist ● Social worker ● Chaplain ● Complementary therapist ● Art therapist ● Music therapist ● Lymphoedema specialist ● Dietician	The hospice or hospice-at-home team provide specialist support in the following: ● Physical care ● Social care ● Psychological care ● Spiritual care ● Domains of assessed care ● Symptom management of complex problems ● Specialist access to services due to end-of-life issues ● Family-support teams (specialist social workers) often deal with social/psychological issues, preparation for bereavement, loss and counselling ● Specialist complementary therapy, art, music, massage, aromatherapy

What makes an interprofessional team an effective team?

As we have already discussed, interprofessional teams come in many shapes and sizes within the health- and social-care sectors, from larger network teams through to smaller individual patient-centred teams. It is important that, whatever the shape and size of the team, the team is effective. The following factors contribute towards effective teamwork.

Clear team goal

It is very difficult to get there if you do not know where you are going!

An effective team will have a shared common goal, which is clear and achievable, providing team members with a focus and direction for their efforts. The goal will have defined outcomes that are measurable, enabling team members to monitor their progress towards successful achievement of their overall goal.

Open communication

Members of effective teams inform each other of who is doing what, when, where and how. Ensuring that relevant information is shared with each team member will enable the team to make the best decisions, thus enhancing the service that the team provide to their patients. Effective teams do not guard information; they share it freely.

Support for innovation

Effective teams work in a climate in which innovation is encouraged and supported by their organisation, with adequate time and resources factored in. Management support for innovation encourages teams to develop new ideas and ways in which to work that will ultimately enhance the morale and thus the output of the team. Research into the effectiveness of health care teams in the NHS (Borrill *et al.*, 2000) has found that teams comprising a mix of professional groups are linked to higher innovation than teams of one group.

High levels of participation

All team members must participate fully in the team's activities if the team is to function well. For this to occur there must be a general climate of trust within the team. Team members should feel 'safe' to contribute ideas, and challenge current practices without fear of recrimination from other team members.

Clear roles and responsibilities

Teams will work more effectively if the roles and responsibilities of team members are clearly articulated and understood by those team members. Misunderstandings and conflicts often occur when roles and expectations are not clearly defined. Awareness among the team of each other's roles and responsibilities will help teams to cope constructively with professional conflicts.

Competent team members

Competent team members are crucial if a team is to work effectively. Equally important is that the team members are placed in the right position. Sometimes, a highly competent professional can be ill-placed, which can upset the team functioning. It is important that problems are dealt with and that if a team member is persistently failing to work with others and targets are not being met, that they are dealt with through the appropriate management and disciplinary procedures.

Effective time management

How a team structures its meetings and meets its deadlines reflects its effectiveness. Teams that manage their meetings well encourage high performance and therefore they have an increased chance of meeting their goals.

Values diversity

The members of an interprofessional health- or social-care team have diverse value systems which can be a key source of interpersonal conflict within a team. However, if a team learns to value each other's differences, they can build on each other's strengths. The overall impact is that individuals appreciate diversity and work together more effectively.

High level of commitment

The effectiveness of a team is associated with a high level of commitment to quality in the team. Commitment to a team is only achieved through all members of the team sharing the same values. This will mean that team members will be motivated to achieve their goals through the provision of a high-quality, innovative service. Team members will enjoy their work, giving them job satisfaction, leading to organisational commitment.

Joint education and training

Work-based learning enables practitioners to learn more effectively together (Barr, 2002). If professionals are learning together, this will encourage and enhance effective interprofessional teamwork. Opportunities for interprofessional education occur at both pre- and post-registration level. The education and learning which may take place is varied: qualificatory courses offered by a university; local/national/international joint conferences/study days; interprofessional training days offered by local service providers; continuing professional development in the practice environment linked to current health- or social-care initiatives.

Effective conflict resolution

Effective teams expect conflicts and differences of opinion, but how the team resolve their conflicts can make or break them. An effective team will focus on the task at hand, not on the individuals in the team, which helps the team move forward and redirect their focus toward positive outcomes.

Moral support and team spirit

Members of effective teams support each other, take pride in and feel loyalty for their teams. The team members will let each other know how they appreciate each other's efforts and ideas and will help each other as and when needed.

Over to you

Working in teams can be rewarding, but at times it is difficult and frustrating. It is just as important to be aware of those factors that can result in a team under-performing as well as those factors that enhance teamwork. Table 3.8 below identifies some of the things that can go wrong in teams. Think about a team in which you are an active member. This could be a work-related team or a team you are involved with in your leisure time, for example a sports team or a musical band. Complete the table below by considering the following:

- Identify those problems which are present in your team and which you feel need most attention.
- For each problem identified, what action could you take to make your team a more effective team?

Table 3.8 What might be going wrong?

Tick	What might be going wrong?	Action to be taken
	Not listening to each other	
	Not clarifying what your objective is	
	Allowing individuals to dominate	
	Allowing individuals to withdraw	
	Not recording what has been decided	
	Not recognising the feelings of members of the team	
	Blaming each other for not meeting deadlines	
	Not clarifying who is going to do what	
	Not clarifying what has to be done by when	
	Not contributing equally to the progress of the team	
	Not being committed to the team	
	Not managing team meetings well	
	Not keeping to agreed practices	
	Not generating new ideas	

RRRRRRapid recap

Check your progress so far by working through each of the following questions.

1. What are the essential features of a team?
2. What are the essential characteristics of teamwork?
3. What are the five stages of team development?
4. List Belbin's nine team roles, which he considered were necessary if a team was to be successful.
5. What factors contribute towards effective interprofessional teamwork?

If you have difficulty with more than one of the questions, read through the section again to refresh your understanding before moving on.

References

Barr, H. (2002) *Interprofessional Education: Today, Yesterday and Tomorrow; A Review.* Available from: www.health.heacademy.ac.uk/publications/occasionalpaper/occp1revised.pdf.

Belbin, R.M. (1981) *Management Teams: Why they Succeed or Fail.* Heinemann, London.

Borrill, C.S., Carletta, J., Carter, A.J., Dawson, J.F., Garrod, S., Rees, R., Richards, A., Shapiro, D. and West, M.A. (2000) *The Effectiveness of Health care Teams in the National Health Service. Final Report.* Available from: www.homepages.inf.ed.ac.uk/jeanc/DOH-final-report.pdf.

Katzenbach, J.R. and Smith, D.K. (1993) *The Wisdom of Teams: Creating the High Performance Organisation.* Harvard Business School Press, Boston, MA.

Kekki, P. (1990) *Teamwork in Primary Care.* World Health Organization, Geneva.

Manion, J., Lorimer, W. and Leander, W.J. (1996) *Team-based Health Care Organisations: Blueprint for Success.* Apsen, Gaithersburg, MD.

Margerison, C.J. and McCann, D. (1995) *Team Management: Practical New* Approaches (2nd ed.). Management Books, Oxford.

Øvretveit, J. (1997) How to Describe Interprofessional Working. In *Interprofessional Working for Health and Social Care* (eds. Øvretveit, J., Mathias, P. and Thomson, T. Macmillan, London, pp. 9–33.

Payne, M. (2000) *Teamwork in Multiprofessional Care.* Palgrave, Basingstoke.

Pritchard, P. and Pritchard, J. (1994) *Teamwork for Primary and Shared Care: A Practical Workbook* (2nd edn). Oxford University Press, Oxford.

Royal Pharmaceutical Society of Great Britain and the British Medical Association (2000) *Teamworking in Primary Health Care: Realising Shared Aims in Patient Care. Final Report.* Royal Pharmaceutical Society of Great Britain and BMA, London. Available from: www.rpsgb.org.uk/pdfs/teamworking.pdf.

Tuckman, B.W. and Jenson, M.A.C. (1977) Stages of Small Group Development Revisited. *Group and Organisational Studies*, **2**: 419–427.

World Health Organization (1978) *Alma Ata 1978 Primary Care.* World Health Organization, Geneva.

4
Leadership and expertise

Learning outcomes

By the end of this chapter you should be able to:

★ Identify the key elements which relate to effective leadership

★ Understand the complex nature of expertise

★ Discuss the relationship between knowledge and expertise

★ Have insight into how expertise influences the leadership within an interprofessional team.

What is leadership?

Leadership . . .

> Go to the people
> Live among them
> Start with what they have
> Build with them
> And, when the deed is done
> The mission accomplished
> The people will say
> 'We have done it ourselves'
>
> Lao Tzu (6th century BC)

Although leadership has been of interest to society for many years, there still appears to be no ultimately authoritative definition of leadership within the literature. Examples of definitions of leadership are given below:

> [a process that] changes both leader and follower
>
> Burns (1978)

> the behaviour of an individual that results in non-coercive influence when that person is directing and co-ordinating the activities of a group toward the accomplishment of a shared goal.
>
> Rowden (2000, p. 30)

> Leadership is the relationship between those who inspire to lead and those who choose to follow.
>
> Kouzes and Posner (2002)

As well as the differing definitions of leadership, the literature reveals that leadership is a complex topic, with the existence of many theories and typologies. Trying to navigate your way through the wealth of literature on leadership could be likened to trying to find your way out of a maze!

The approach taken to leadership in this chapter will be to trace the developments in ideas of leadership and to discuss the significance of those developments to interprofessional leadership and interprofessional working.

Early research into leadership was concerned with identifying traits of leadership, so that the people with the right traits could be selected for leadership roles. The so-called 'trait theory' was based on the premise that leaders are born rather than created. Stogdhill (1974) identified traits and skills considered to be essential to a successful leader.

Table 4.1 Traits and skills of a successful leader

Traits	Skills
• Adaptable to situations	• Intelligent
• Ambitious and achievement oriented	• Creative
• Dependable	• Diplomatic and tactful
• Energetic	• Organised
• Self-confident	• Persuasive
• Willing to take responsibility	• Socially skilled
• Persistent	• Conceptually skilled
• Dominant	• Knowledgeable about group task
• Assertive	• Articulate
• Cooperative	
• Decisive	
• Tolerant of stress	

However, early researchers began to identify problems with the trait theory. For example, this approach did not look at whether the leaders were effective or not and it is also difficult to identify whether individuals have the required traits or not. As a result, researchers turned their attention to what leaders did, that is, how they behaved, especially towards their followers (team members). Researchers, therefore, moved from studying the leaders to studying leadership. There was recognition that leadership was a behavioural pattern that could be learned. Different patterns of behaviour were grouped together and labelled as leadership styles. The following section discusses these leadership styles.

Leadership styles

A number of different leadership styles emerged from these studies, which were based on different assumptions and theories. The style that a leader adopts is based on their beliefs, values and preferences as well as the organisational cultures and norms around them. Different organisations will encourage some styles while discouraging others. The following leadership styles will be considered:

1. Participative leadership
2. Situational leadership
3. Transactional leadership
4. Transformational leadership
5. Charismatic leadership.

Participative leadership

A participative leader, as the name suggests, is a leader who actively involves other people in the decision-making process, for example team members, peers, managers and appropriate stakeholders. The level of involvement that others have in the decision-making process will vary depending on the preferences and beliefs of the leader and the type of decision being made.

Table 4.2 Spectrum of participation

Not participative				Highly participative
Autocratic decision by leader	Leader proposes decision, listens to feedback and then decides	Team proposes decision, leader has final decision	Joint decision with team as equals	Full delegation of decision to team

Advantages of this style of leadership include:

*   team members are more committed to decisions if they have been involved in the decision-making process
*   involvement in decision-making improves the team members, understanding of the issues involved
*   team members deciding together make better decisions than one person alone.

Participative leadership is not without its critics and its main problem is one shared with the trait theory. Researchers often did not consider the context or setting in which the leadership style was being used. For example, advocates of participative leadership assumed that the same style of leadership would work as well in a team of footballers as in an accident and emergency department.

Situational leadership

As researchers realised that both the environment and the abilities of the team members significantly influenced the style that the leader adopted, researchers began to turn their attention to these two factors. A number of models emerged which were based on the interaction of the characteristics of the leader, the characteristics of the followers, and the situation. One of the more influential models that emerged is the one developed by Hersey and Blanchard (1977).

This model identified four leadership styles that could be selected to deal with contrasting situations. The style that the leader chose depended upon the amount and support that the leader needed to give to an individual team leader.

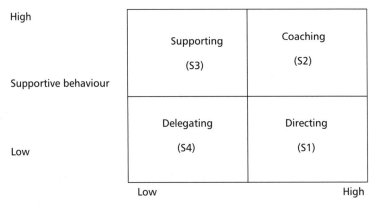

Figure 4.1 Hersey and Blanchard's four leadership styles

Directing (S1)

The leader defines the roles and tasks of the team members and supervises closely. The leader makes the decisions and tells the team members, so communication is largely one way. This style of leadership might be used when a new member joins the team, or where a task has to be completed within a very short time span.

Coaching (S2)

The leader still defines the roles and tasks, but seeks ideas and suggestions from the team member. The leader still makes the decision but communication is much more two way.

Supporting (S3)

The leader gives day-to-day decisions to the team member. The leader facilitates and takes part in the decisions, but control is with the team member.

Delegating (S4)

The leader is still involved in decisions and problem solving but the control is with the team member.

An effective leader will be versatile and will be able to move around the four leadership styles depending on the situation. There is no one right style but a leader will have a preferred style. As previously stated, the style adopted by the leader will not only depend on the situation but also on the characteristics of the individual team member. To take this into account, Hersey and Blanchard (1977) identified four development levels, which, like the leadership styles, varied depending on the situation. The four development levels are as follows:

- **D1** – Generally lacking the specific skills required for the task and lacks confidence and/or motivation.
- **D2** – May have some of the relevant skills, but will be unable to do the task without some support. The task or situation may be new to them.
- **D3** – Experienced and capable, but may lack confidence to do it without support or the motivation to do it well.
- **D4** – Experienced at the job/task and comfortable with their ability to do it well.

D3	High competence	D2	Some competence
	Variable commitment		Low commitment
S3	Supporting	S2	Coaching
D4	High competence	D1	Low competence
	High commitment		Low commitment
S4	Delegating	S1	Directing

Figure 4.2 *The relationship between the four leadership styles and the four development levels of the team member*

The key feature of a situational leadership model, like the Hersey and Blanchard (1977) model, is that if a leader selects a style that is suited to the context and to the ability of the team member, the leader and consequently the team will be more successful. There are, however, limitations with such a model which include:

- The model mainly focuses on the relationship between leaders and their team members and does not consider issues of organisational structure, politics, economics and professional socialisation.
- The model does not take into account cultural factors. Cultural factors influence the way people carry out, and respond to, different leadership styles.

Reflective activity

A senior practitioner joins your team and you are asked to look after him during his first few days.

With reference to this scenario consider the following:

- think about what the senior practitioner needs to know/find out in the first few days in your team
- for each task identified, use Hersey and Blanchard's (1977) model to select the appropriate style of leadership
- think about the benefits and drawbacks for both you and your colleague of adopting the style of leadership that you have selected for each task.

Transactional leadership

Transactional leadership is built on a system of give and take, with the relationship between the leader and the follower being developed from the exchange of rewards and promises for the effort put in by the follower, for example salary increase, attendance at study days/conferences, recognition, praise. The leader clarifies goals and objectives, communicates, and organises tasks and activities for their team members to ensure that the specified goals of the team are met (Burns, 1978). This style of leadership is hierarchical and is a reactive, as opposed to proactive, style of leadership, in that it deals with day-to-day activities and issues. It has been found that this style of leadership is more evident in first-level managers, than in high-level managers (Avolio and Bass, 1988). A first-level manager would be a practitioner who is leading other practitioners in the day-to-day delivery of care to patients/clients. An example of a first-level manager would be a senior therapeutic radiographer, responsible for the day-to-day running of a treatment unit in an oncology department. The senior radiographer would have responsibilities including scheduling of patients, treatment delivery, ensuring that the team all have coffee and lunch breaks and problem solving. As a first-level manager's primary role is operational rather than strategic, it is not surprising that first-level managers have a tendency to adopt a transactional style of leadership. First-level managers also usually work in an environment that is conducive to a transactional leadership style. The type of environment where transactional leadership may prevail is in routine situations where the basic level of anxiety is not high and where there is no acute sense of impending crisis or major change (Popper and Zakkai, 1994).

Despite much research that highlights the limitations of transactional leadership, this is a popular approach that is still used today.

Transformational and charismatic leadership styles are also currently popular. It is these leadership styles that are used in the leadership development programmes that are aimed at leaders working in the health sector. These two styles of leadership are discussed in the following two sections.

Transformational leadership

The foundation of transformational leadership rests on the four behaviours that were identified by Bass (1985). These four behaviours, also referred to as the four I's of transformational leadership (Bass and Avolio, 1994), comprise of three factors:

1. **I**dealised influence/**I**nspirational motivation.
2. **I**ntellectual stimulation.
3. **I**ndividual consideration.

Idealised influence/inspirational motivation (Bass and Avolio, 1994)

These two behaviours go together and behaviours associated with idealised influence/inspirational motivation include:

- instilling pride in and among the team
- talking optimistically about the future
- encouraging followers to go beyond self-interest for the good of the group
- articulating a vision for the future which is exciting
- providing reassurance that obstacles can be overcome
- encouraging confidence in achieving and carrying out goals and tasks.

Intellectual stimulation (Bass and Avolio, 1994)

This is characterised by encouraging intelligence, consistency, logical thinking and careful problem solving. The behaviours associated with intellectual stimulation include:

- actively seeking different perspectives when solving problems
- suggesting new ways of looking at completing tasks
- encouraging rethinking of ideas that have not been questioned in the past.

Individual consideration (Bass and Avolio, 1994)

Individual consideration is concerned with the leader treating the followers as individuals and not just as members of the group. Behaviours related to individual consideration include:

- spending time teaching and coaching
- helping others develop their strengths
- actively listening to others' concerns.

If we put these four behaviour types together then we start to build a picture of what a transformational leader 'looks like'. Below is an account of what a transformational leader might look like and feel like for their followers.

A transformational leader is concerned with change and action, in other words they are visionary. They put passion and energy into everything they do and in doing so they engage the hearts and minds of others. This style of leadership requires facilitation and concern for the individual team members.

Transformational leaders develop a clear collective vision that will excite and enthuse their team members and they communicate it effectively to their team members. The leader takes every opportunity to 'sell' the vision to their team, encouraging team members to commit to the vision. Trust and personal integrity are central features of the relationship that the leader has with the followers. It is through the followers' trust and respect in their leader that the followers are motivated to perform beyond expectation (Shamir *et al.*, 1994).

A transformational leader is always visible and by acting as role models, they inspire team members to put the good of the whole team above self-interest. The leader encourages team members to be more innovative and is prepared, him- or herself, to take personal risk. It is the leader's unwavering commitment that keeps the team members going, particularly when the team begins to believe that the vision can never be achieved.

Transformational leaders coach and mentor team members, encouraging them to develop both personally and professionally. They care about individual team members and want them to succeed.

When the benefits of transformational leadership for the team are considered, it is perhaps not surprising that this style of leadership is frequently used in leadership development programmes within health- and social-care settings. The benefits of transformational leadership include:

- significant increases in team performance
- higher commitment to the team from individual team members
- increased trust in the leader from team members
- enhanced team-member satisfaction with both their job and the leader
- reduced team-member stress and increased wellbeing
- enhanced quality of the services the team provide.

Transactional and transformational leadership

These two styles of leadership (both discussed above) are not mutually exclusive. In transformational leadership, the power of the leader comes from creating understanding and trust and facilitating. While transformational leadership creates a high-performance culture within a team, elements of transactional leadership are required to ensure a clear focus on the achievement and measurement of results. This would suggest that an effective leader will be able to combine the two styles, so that targets, results and procedures are delivered by developing shared understanding and commitment.

If the benefits of transformational leadership are coupled with the benefits of transactional leadership, it is clear that this combination of leadership style would be particularly suitable for interprofessional team leaders. Table 4.3 illustrates features of an interpersonal team that make it suitable for a transformational/transactional style of leadership.

Table 4.3 Interprofessional team features and leadership styles

Interprofessional team feature	Leadership style
Day-to-day activities and tasks need to be achieved, for example the care of a specific patient/client.	Transactional
The team will need to work within the structures and boundaries of the organisation.	Transactional
The team is usually non-hierarchical, with the different professionals all working towards the same goals.	Transformational
The team will have a long-term vision, which will be driven by government papers and policies.	Transformational
The development needs of the individual team member are paramount, not only for the personal and professional development of the individual but also to the development of the team as a whole.	Transformational
Team members are often working autonomously within an interprofessional team and therefore it is essential that they are empowered to control themselves and to manage their own problem solving.	Transformational

Over to you

Look at this website:
www.rcn.org.uk/resources/practicedevelopment/about-pd/processes/leadership/
Read the article titled 'Transformational Leadership processes'. This article provides a useful summary for those interested in developing transformational leadership skills.

Charismatic leadership (Conger and Kanungo, 1988, 1998)

Charismatic leadership is a relatively recently studied style of leadership. The development of this style of leadership is related to the type of environment that many organisations find themselves operating within in the 21st century. Today, many organisations, including the health- and social care sectors, work in environments which are high risk, highly unpredictable and where there are rapid and often major changes taking place. These situations are characterised by high levels of anxiety and uncertainty that intensify processes of attribution, projection and transference and increase a perceived need for a charismatic leader. The charismatic leader is an image created by the followers, who use the leader as a 'screen' for their projections and attributions (Popper and Zakkai, 1994).

Conger and Kanungo (1998) identified five behaviours that are exhibited by charismatic leaders, these are:

1. Can articulate a vision.

2. Show sensitivity to members' needs.

3. Show environmental sensitivity.

4. Exhibit unconventional behaviour.

5. Take personal risks.

If these are the characteristics that a charismatic leader exhibits, what does a charismatic leader 'look' like? A charismatic leader uses their charm and personality to empower team members to believe in their own ability and to internalise the leader's vision before accepting it as their own. If this happens, it is likely that the leader will get their team members' respect. This style of leader will often deliver simple rather than complex visions.

A charismatic leader will show a great deal of interest in the team member that they are talking to at that moment, making the team member feel like they are, for that time, the most important person in the world. This type of leader is very perceptive and will be able to pick up on the moods and concerns of not only the individual team members but also the team as a whole. This enables the leader to focus their action and words to suit the situation at that moment in time.

A charismatic leader characteristically has a high level of self-belief, and will show enormous confidence in their team members. They are very persuasive and engender trust through taking personal risks in the name of their beliefs.

From the description thus far, it would appear that a charismatic leader possesses similar skills and attributes to those of a transformational leader. There is, however, one fundamental difference between the two styles of leadership and that is their basic focus. A transformational leader's focus is transforming the team and their team members, whereas a charismatic leader may not want to change anything, and may be more concerned with him- or herself than anyone else.

There are some drawbacks to a charismatic leader:

● they have a tendency to dominate

● they tend to prefer the 'big picture' to the detriment of the day-to-day operational detail of their vision

● their motives and strategies may not always be ethical

- team leaders become over reliant and dependant on their leader. If there is too much admiration the leader may feel that they are infallible. It is crucial that team members do not get swept along in a wave of enthusiasm created by their leader without stopping and questioning/re-examining the vision. Just because the leader believes something is right, it does not of course mean that it is right
- they do not usually train and develop their successors and thus there is no natural successor if they leave the team or organisation
- they may be narcissistic and need power to cover their low self-esteem and possible lack of certain essential leadership skills. This potential lack of skills in a charismatic leader can be disastrous for the leader and their team members.

What makes an effective team leader?

There is no doubt that the way in which a team is led will have a major impact upon the success or otherwise of the team. We are all able to identify a 'good' and a 'not so good' team leader, but what skills and behaviour does the team leader possess or not possess that leads us to make that decision?

Reflective activity

Consider the skills, behaviour and qualities that you think make a good team leader.

 Case study

Leading a team

Maggie, a lead diagnostic radiographer is responsible for the day-to-day management of the CT Scanner. Her responsibilities include coordinating the workflow and directing a multidisciplinary team. The team includes at least one other senior radiographer with some skill and experience; a training radiographer; a student radiographic assistant; a radiologist who oversees the list and who is available for interventional procedures (biopsy/drainage), with a nurse as support. In addition, Maggie has to liaise closely with reception staff, secretarial staff (within the CT/medical imaging department), referring clinicians, ward staff and portering staff.

Maggie acts as a role model, providing strong clinical leadership underpinned by sound clinical practice, to promote a professional and smooth-running service (an effective and efficient service). She has the skills, knowledge, expertise and experience and furthermore the confidence, sense of responsibility, motivation and independence to deal with all situations within her department.

Maggie assesses the ability and willingness of the individuals within her team and adopts different leadership styles appropriate to the situation to encourage the members of her team to grow in all areas of their job.

continued

Julie, a first-year student diagnostic radiographer, has just arrived as a new member of the team. As it is only her second day in the department, Maggie tells Julie what needs to be done. She gives very detailed instructions and supervises her closely to ensure that the tasks are being carried out correctly. For example, she asks Julie to help the patients change into a patient gown before their scans; collect the films from the processor; and assign them to the correct film packet ready for the radiologist to report.

Maggie also has a third-year diagnostic radiography student, Peter, in her team. Peter has experience of working in the CT scanning department and is keen to learn and willing to take responsibility. Maggie still gives him a lot of support and direction, but seeks Peter's involvement in the task, discussing the task with him, why it is necessary, how it can be best done.

James is the senior radiographer within Maggie's team. Maggie is able to allow him to take full responsibility for his work. She is, of course, there in the background to support James should that become necessary.

With reference to the case study:

- What type of leadership style do you think Maggie has adopted for Julie, Peter and James?
- What leadership skills do you think Maggie has?
- Are there any other skills that Maggie needs to effectively lead her multidisciplinary team?
- What do you think is Maggie's vision for her team?
- Is the structure of Maggie's team hierarchical or horizontal?

In an attempt to draw together the qualities that an effective leader would require, the *NHS Leadership Qualities Framework* will be discussed. Recognising that leaders in health- and social care were grappling with an enormous agenda for change (for example, *Agenda for Change*, the Knowledge and Skills Framework, new ways of working and new roles), the NHS Leadership Centre, published the *NHS Leadership Qualities Framework* (Department of Health, 2002) to help NHS staff to analyse their leadership roles and responsibilities. The Framework was researched and developed over a two-year period by the Hay Group in consultation with leaders within the service.

The *NHS Leadership Qualities Framework* (Department of Health, 2002) comprises of 15 leadership qualities (characteristics, attitudes and behaviours), which can be used to identify both effective and outstanding leaders. These leadership qualities have been grouped into three clusters.

Cluster one: personal qualities

- Self-belief
- Self-awareness
- Self-management
- Drive for improvement
- Personal integrity.

Cluster two: setting direction

- Seizing the future
- Intellectual flexibility
- Broad scanning
- Political awareness
- Drive for results.

Cluster three: delivering the service

- Leading change through people
- Holding to account
- Empowering others
- Effective and strategic influencing
- Collaborative working.

If we review the qualities identified above, it is possible to see that the majority of them can be found in the leadership styles described in the previous section, in participative, situational, transactional, transformational and charismatic styles.

Evidence base

Go onto the website www.nhsleadershipqualities.nhs.uk/ and read the *NHS Leadership Qualities Framework*. This document provides full details of the Framework, including how to implement the framework within your organisation, and also provides a useful set of scenarios for understanding the combination of qualities that effective leaders use in particular settings.

Key points | Top tips

Effective leaders:

- possess qualities such as honesty, integrity, humility, courage, commitment, confidence, passion, determination and sensitivity
- make deliberate choices about how to tackle different situations and people
- do best when they adopt leadership styles that express their personality preferences and allow them to play to their strengths
- support the developmental needs of their individual team members
- are able to assess the competence levels of their team members and their commitment to completing tasks to achieve the required outcomes
- are able to balance the demands of the day-to-day tasks and team dynamics so that the needs of everyone involved in completing the task are taken into account
- have a vision and are able to motivate and inspire people to put the vision into practice
- want to make a real difference to people's health by delivering high-quality services and by developing the services provided by the team to patients and clients
- have a high level of self-awareness and know their own strengths and limitations.

What is an expert?

As health- and social-care practitioners, we often remark that Sally or Julie or Imran are 'expert' practitioners and that we would be happy for that particular practitioner to care for us or a member of our family. But what makes an 'expert' practitioner, how do we know when we have seen one and why, in the context of interprofessional working, is it important to be able to define an expert practitioner? Using a case-study approach, we will discuss the issues raised by these questions.

Health professional speaks

Two health care professionals were asked the same question related to their own profession:

What is an 'expert'?

Anja, a therapeutic radiographer, gave the following response:

Knowledgeable, I think it's important to know things like side-effects, knowledge about a machine if you see something that's going a bit wrong, you can pick up minor faults before problems occur, knowledge on x-rays. I think an expert is organised, a team player, a good communicator so that they can communicate with the team and with patients as well, accurate, flexible and motivated. I also think that an expert has the confidence of experience, professionalism, technical ability, it's that judgement based upon experience, but still being able to treat that patient as an individual. It's knowing how far to go when and with what type of patient. For example, some patients like having your arm to lead them into the treatment room, while others might be offended by it, it's that judgement.

I think you can always tell your junior staff from senior staff in the way that they can deal with things. I think radiographers all have a lesson plan, perhaps a young-person lesson plan, a child lesson plan, an old-person lesson plan and even a patient-with-a-bladder-tumour lesson plan, because they've been there, it's an acceptable lesson plan and they're able to respond to those cues coming from the patient quickly. It's the adaptability, it's the expert element.

Suresh, a mental-health nurse, gave this response:

You want to know how an 'expert' mental-health nurse can be recognised? It's tempting to try and be funny but this is a serious question and not easy to answer. It is too obvious to say that this is a person who uses advanced knowledge, skill, education and experience in practice, although that is important. Alternatively, I could talk about their ability to establish an effective therapeutic alliance with the other. Um, no. Humanists would talk about the attributes of the complete person. Not terribly helpful.

I think the expert can be distinguished by the economic, skilful and smooth way in which they establish therapeutic alliances within their professional role. The expert mental-health nurse negotiates, with the client and themselves, about the purpose and activity of the relationship. They draw upon an extensive repertoire of skill and depth of experiential and theoretical knowledge. They don't always bring to conscious thought the whole of the decision-making process because some conclusions are less reasoned than intuitively known.

I believe that they operate in the most appropriate place on several scales:
Considered . . . . spontaneous
Self-disclosing . . . . private
Expressive . . . . controlled

Also they avoid façades yet can function within required social roles, they have a healthy respect and liking for themselves that they extend to others. I also think that they have a childlike and warm sense of humour and engage with the other as person.

Professional knowledge

As the concept of knowledge features prominently in Anja and Suresh's accounts, we will begin our exploration of expertise by discussing what is meant by professional knowledge.

The nature of professional knowledge is complex and it is difficult to define its exact nature. This should not, however, prevent us from attempting to tease out the essential meaning of professional knowledge. In this section, we will explore the various types of knowledge that make up the strands of professional knowledge.

Oakeshott (1962, cited in Eraut, 1994) makes a clear distinction between 'technical knowledge' and 'practical knowledge'. Technical knowledge, he suggests, is capable of written codification, that is, knowledge that can be articulated in the written form, for example in textbooks. Practical knowledge, on the other hand, is expressed only in practice and learned only through experience of practice. Practical knowledge has traditionally not been capable of written codification. Intuition and professional judgement are examples of practical knowledge.

Patel *et al.* (1999) state that there are two basic types of knowledge: knowledge that can be verbalised, such as knowledge of facts and concepts; and knowledge that cannot be verbalised, such as intuition and knowledge of procedures. These two types of knowledge are referred to as propositional knowledge and non-propositional knowledge respectively.

Other authors have used different labels for these two types of knowledge, Ryle (1949) called them 'knowing that' and' knowing how', and Anderson (1983) referred to them as declarative knowledge and procedural knowledge.

Table 4.4 How authors have classified the two main types of knowledge

Author	Knowledge that can be verbalised, e.g. facts	Knowledge which cannot be verbalised, e.g. intuition
Ryle (1949)	'Knowing that'	'Knowing how'
Anderson (1983)	Declarative knowledge	Procedural knowledge
Oakeshott (cited in Eraut, 1994)	Technical knowledge	Practical knowledge
Patel *et al.* (1999)	Propositional knowledge	Non-propositional knowledge

If we look at the 'Health Professional Speaks' feature on pages 68–69, we can see that both Anja and Suresh talk about these two different types of knowledge. Anja talks about experts needing knowledge of side-effects, x-rays and treatment machines. All of this knowledge can be found in a textbook and is, therefore, propositional knowledge.

Both Anja and Suresh refer to non-propositional knowledge. Suresh talks about experts not always bringing to conscious thought the whole of the decision-making process because some decisions are intuitively known. Anja mentions 'judgement based on experience' and practice being 'implied' rather than 'seen'. This suggests that Anja is distinguishing between the two types of knowledge, 'implied' referring to non- propositional knowledge and 'seen' referring to propositional knowledge.

Personal knowledge is another strand of professional knowledge. Everyone acquires knowledge through experiences, either directly or vicariously, much of which does not have much apparent connection with learning. This type of knowledge has been referred to as personal knowledge (Kolb, 1984; Eraut, 1994; Fish, 1998). Many of the experiences we have are simply lived through unless the 'act of attention' halts the process and confers a meaning on the experience. When attention is focused more deeply upon an experience, it can be understood in a meaningful way. One important way in which health- and social-care practitioners 'halt' this process, and thus give meaning to their experiences, is by reflecting on their practice.

However, personal knowledge is not created in a vacuum but is constructed through interaction with the social, political, economical and cultural context in which the experience occurs. This latter knowledge is referred to a social knowledge, which Kolb defines as:

> independent, socially and culturally transmitted networks of
> words, symbols and images based solely on comprehension
>
> Kolb (1984, p. 105)

Personal knowledge and social knowledge can be seen as complementary, with an individual's development being the product of the transaction between personal experience and the system of social knowledge interacted with.

Vygotsky's (1978) work emphasises the societal context of an individual's cognitive development. Central to his theory is the concept of the 'zone of proximal development', in which a novice's development occurs through participation in activities slightly beyond their competence with the assistance of more skilled practitioners. Learning takes place in the zone of proximal development via interactions between an individual's personal knowledge system and the society within which the learning is taking place.

For the purposes of description, it may be easy to separate out the different types of knowledge: propositional knowledge; non-propositional knowledge; personal knowledge; social knowledge, but during practice the different types of knowledge are inextricably linked. As Williams succinctly states:

> During professional action, knowledge becomes a dynamic integrated 'whole' which is shaped and adapted to fit each situation which is encountered.
>
> Williams (1998, p. 29)

Professional knowledge is not a discrete entity and undoubtedly the development of professional knowledge is affected by the social, cultural, historical, attitudinal, psychological and behavioural context that the individual is operating within. However, making practical knowledge more explicit and thus accessible for codification, criticism and dissemination would help to enhance understanding of the nature of expertise, in the health- and social-care professions. Also when working within an interprofessional team, it is important that practitioners are able to make their practical knowledge accessible to others in the team. In this way practitioners will be able to appreciate, for example, how and why individual members of the team arrive at specific decisions or problem-solve in a particular way. An important part of this process is to be able to define what makes an 'expert' practitioner.

Key points Top tips

The strands of professional knowledge are:

- propositional knowledge
- non-propositional knowledge
- personal knowledge
- social knowledge

Experience and expertise

If we look back again at the 'Health professional speaks' feature on page 68 we can see that Anja and Suresh have used the word 'experience' to describe an important characteristic of an expert practitioner in their field of practice. But what does 'experience' actually mean and how does it forward an understanding of what an expert practitioner is? As the concept of experience features prominently in Anja and Suresh's accounts and also within the literature on expertise, it would suggest that an understanding of the nature of experience would be useful when defining an expert. The definition of 'experience' is often taken for granted, yet there appears to be no agreement within the literature as to what constitutes an experience (Boud *et al.*, 1993). A dictionary definition of 'experience' does not encapsulate the holistic nature of experience but breaks it into its component parts, for example 'direct personal participation or observation', 'a particular incident, feeling etc., that a person has undergone', 'accumulated knowledge, especially of practical matters' (*The Collins Dictionary and Thesaurus*, 1989). Oakeshott (1933, cited in Boud *et al.*, 1993, p. 9) sees experience as having two elements, 'experiencing' and 'what is experienced', and that these two elements compose a single whole.

Kolb makes the following comments about experience:

> The transactional relationship between the person and the environment . . . symbolised in the dual meanings of the term experience – one subjective and personal referring to the person's internal state . . . and the other objective and environmental
>
> Kolb (1984, p. 35)

Boud *et al.* (1993, p. 9) characterise experience as having 'within it judgement, thought and connectedness with other experience – it is not isolated'. This definition suggests that experience is a meaningful encounter.

Ericsson (1996, p. 9) makes reference to a '10-year rule of preparation' before an individual becomes an expert in their chosen domain. To support this rule, Ericsson (1996) cites a number of studies: Simon and Chase (1973), who suggested that no one became a grand master in chess in fewer than nine to 10 years, and Patel *et al.* (1996) who speak of the necessity of 10 years' preparation before a doctor can call themselves an expert.

Clearly, experience is important for the achievement of expertise, but it is the nature of this accrued experience that will determine whether an individual will become an expert. The simple accumulation of practice is not sufficient; if you endlessly repeat the same exercise, you will not develop into an expert. Time must be accompanied by the chance to accumulate a varied set of meaningful experiences.

Models for developing expertise

Various models for developing expertise can be found within the literature. This section will describe two of these models:

1. The Dreyfus model of skill acquisition (Dreyfus and Dreyfus, 1986).
2. The cognitive continuum theory (Hammond, 1980).

It is important to discuss these models of expertise as they provide an insight into the way in which an expert practitioner develops. These models highlight that an interprofessional team will have practitioners not only from different professions but also at different stages of their development, in other words, practitioners will have more or less expertise in their field than other practitioners within their team.

Dreyfus and Dreyfus (1986) model of skill acquisition

This model has as its key contextual feature, experience. Hubert Dreyfus, a philosopher, and Stuart Dreyfus, an operations researcher, describe a five-stage model for the development of expertise. An individual must go through each stage to become an expert in their domain, the five stages being novice, advanced beginner, competent, proficient and expert. The movement from novice to expert relies upon the practitioner accumulating situated practical experience and is characterised by the use of intuitive thinking as opposed to analytical thinking and the ability of the practitioner to see a situation as a whole rather than just its individual parts.

Evidence base

Go onto the website www.gp-training.net/training/theory/skill.htm and read about the Dreyfus and Dreyfus (1986) model of skill acquisition. This website provides descriptors for each of the five levels of skill acquisition.

As already stated, experience is the key feature of this model. It is the practitioner's experience with a particular task that determines the cognitive mode selected; for example, a novice is by definition unfamiliar with the task and will adopt an analytic, step-by-step approach. As the novice gains more experience and becomes an advanced beginner, a competent practitioner and then a proficient practitioner, the balance between analytical and intuitive thinking alters so that by the time a practitioner becomes an expert all decisions pertaining to a particular task are carried out intuitively. Dreyfus and Dreyfus state:

> An expert generally knows what to do based on mature and practical understanding . . . an expert's skill has become so much part of him that he need be no more aware of it than he is of his own body . . . when things are proceeding normally experts don't solve problems and don't make decisions; they do what normally works.
>
> (1986, p. 30–31)

A criticism of the Dreyfus and Dreyfus model is the difficulty in applying the five levels of expertise. Practitioners rarely perform at the same level on all tasks in a domain. For example, a therapeutic radiographer may perform at the level of expert when performing tasks that they frequently encounter, for example, discussing with patients the acute side-effects that may result from the radiotherapy treatment they are about to receive. Whereas, they may perform at the level of proficiency for tasks they encounter less frequently, for example 'setting up' patients suffering from cancer of the head and neck region, localising and planning radiotherapy treatments. For tasks that are relatively unfamiliar, for example the application of specialised techniques, the therapeutic radiographer would perform at the level of competence. So it would be a mistake to label a particular therapeutic radiographer as an expert and expect them to perform consistently at that level in all tasks in the domain of therapeutic radiography. A more accurate definition of an expert would be an individual who was capable of handling a wide range of tasks intuitively, compared to an individual with less experience.

Another criticism of the Dreyfus and Dreyfus model is that it claims that novices only think analytically and that experts only think intuitively. Dreyfus and Dreyfus (1986) argue that, because novices are unfamiliar with the task, they have to take an analytical approach. But you could argue that the unfamiliarity of the task induces intuition because the novice has not learnt any analytic principles for organising their thinking about the situation, and thus have to rely on the intuitive method for integrating information (Hamm, 1999).

The Dreyfus and Dreyfus model fails, therefore, to recognise the crucial role that the task plays in influencing the individual to select the appropriate cognitive mode.

Cognitive continuum theory (Hammond, 1980)

This model of expertise, developed by the psychologist Kenneth Hammond, recognises the important role that the task plays in the development of expertise. This theory has three elements; a cognitive continuum, a task continuum and a range of modes of practice. Unlike the Dreyfus and Dreyfus model, which speaks of two pure types of cognition, analytical for novices and intuitive for experts, Hammond (1980) believes that analytical and intuitive thinking should be placed on the poles of a continuum. This is because most thinking is neither purely analytical nor purely intuitive but lies somewhere in between.

The cognitive continuum is of little value to the practitioner if there is no indication as to which kind of thinking to use in various situations. Therefore, to enable the practitioner to convert the idea of the cognitive continuum into guidance about how to think, the task becomes important. The task continuum ranges from analysis-inducing to intuition-inducing and the position that a task occupies on the continuum depends on the type of task, for example the complexity of the task, the ambiguity of the task content and the form of task presentation (Hamm, 1999). Thus, the cognitive continuum theory recognises that it is possible for an expert to think analytically in one situation and intuitively in another depending on the type of task. Dreyfus and Dreyfus claim, conversely, that being an expert means that the individual must take an intuitive approach to all tasks within their domain.

This last point raises another question. If an individual uses intuitive cognition to make decisions, will a greater degree of accuracy be achieved than if analytical cognition is used? Hammond (1980) argues that it is not the mode of cognition that affects the accuracy of a decision, but whether the appropriate mode of cognition has been selected for the task. For example, if the conditions of a task suggest that an analytical approach should be adopted but the individual tries to use an intuitive approach, then errors can occur. Conversely, if the task suggests that an intuitive approach should be adopted and the individual tries to use an analytic approach, then poor performance may result (Hamm, 1999). The evidence suggests that experts perform by way of a variety of cognitive modes, depending on the task, and that this variation is good because an expert's intuition is not infallible in all situations.

Neither the Dreyfus and Dreyfus model nor the cognitive continuum theory has attempted to explain how an individual becomes an expert, only that experience, type of task and modes of cognition have a role in the development of an expert.

Knowledge and expertise

In this section we consider the relationship between knowledge and expertise. Research into expertise has focused on differences between individuals varying in levels of expertise, in terms of memory, reasoning strategies and the role of domain-specific knowledge.

Anja and Suresh, as already discussed in the 'Health professional speaks' feature on page 68, both make reference to knowledge and expertise in their practice. It may appear to be stating the obvious that there is a link between knowledge base and expertise. However, what is important is not only having an extensive body of knowledge but that the knowledge is organised in such a way that it is accessible and useable.

The way in which knowledge is represented in memory has a not insignificant role to play in the differences observed in problem solving by experts and novices. Research has indicated that experts appear to have the following characteristics: experts use forward reasoning to problem solve, whereas novices try to solve problems in a backward way (Simon and Simon, 1978); experts take a more direct route to problem solving than novices (Patel *et al.*, 1994) and that experts problem solve faster and more economically than novices (Chi *et al.*, 1988; Schmidt *et al.*, 1990).

The notion of 'schemes of experience' (Schutz, 1967), frames (Minsky, 1977), scripts (Schank and Abelson, 1977), templates (Boreham, 1988) and illness scripts (Schmidt *et al.*, 1990) will be used to explore these differences in problem solving between novices and experts. Although all of these schemata are subtly different, they all have the same underlying principle, that is, they:

> attempt to describe how acquired knowledge is organised and represented and how such cognitive structures facilitate the use of knowledge in particular ways.
>
> Glaser (1984, p. 100)

Schmidt *et al.*'s (1990) four-stage model of medical expertise recognises that personal experience as well as propositional knowledge has an important role in the development of what Schmidt *et al.* (1990) refer to as 'illness scripts', which are developed during stage three of this model. The clinical experience of the medical practitioner becomes increasingly important during stage three, when illness scripts are being developed, and stage four, when memories of previous patients are being maintained. Stage one is solely concerned with the gaining of knowledge and its development into a network with links made between related pieces of information. It is stage two that is particularly important in the context of this discussion. Stage two involves the transformation of the networks developed by medical students in stage one into abridged networks using high-level causal models, with information about signs and symptoms being subsumed under 'diagnostic labels'. Thus, the medical student is now able to represent a disease in their memory, for example bowel cancer, as opposed to seeing the disease as its individual signs and symptoms, for example diarrhoea, rectal bleeding, pain and so on. As the medical student has had more practical experience, it is possible for them to select only the most critical information and to disregard the irrelevant information to solve a problem.

The idea that performance improves when the individual has access to multiple experiences/stories is important in relation to an expert's superior problem-solving capacities. During stage three of Schmidt *et al.*'s model, 'illness scripts' are developed and these illness scripts provide the medical practitioner with multiple experiences/stories, which they can use when making medical diagnoses. The development of illness scripts is dependant on accumulated experience of working with patients and thus this also supports the generally accepted view that substantial experience is required for expert performance. During stage four, the medical practitioner stores memories of previous patients and, therefore, during stages three and four medical practitioners accumulate numerous rich schemata which they can draw upon to problem solve.

Schemata such as those developed by Schmidt *et al.*'s model go some way to explaining why experts take a more direct route to problem solving compared to novices. The more experienced a practitioner is, the greater the number of schemata they will have accumulated and the more able they will be to use forward reasoning as a problem-solving strategy. For example, if a therapeutic radiographer has seen the same physical and psychological effects arising from treating a patient with a tumour of the pelvic region many times, for example diarrhoea, nausea and vomiting, anxiety, loss of self-esteem and so on, then they are more likely to recognise important cues that will lead more directly to a solution the next time this situation is encountered.

Anja's case study (see 'Health professional speaks' feature on page 68) illustrates this point by reference to the range of 'lesson plans' that therapeutic radiographers have developed through experience.

The 'lesson plans' which Anja refers to appear to be serving the same function as 'illness scripts'.

As schema theory assumes that there are schemata for recurrent situations, then one of the major functions of these schemata will be to construct interpretations of situations, such as those just described. A novice therapeutic radiographer, who by definition will have less accumulated knowledge and therefore fewer schemata to draw upon, will have to think through the problem more explicitly and make more inferences before arriving at a correct solution to the problem.

In conclusion, researchers have taken two different approaches to defining an expert. Models of expertise have been developed, for example the model of skill acquisition (Dreyfus and Dreyfus, 1986), the four-stage model of clinical expertise (Schmidt *et al.*, 1990) and the cognitive continuum theory (Hammond, 1980). These models, however, do not explain how an individual becomes an expert. The second approach appears to address the 'how' by identifying characteristics of an expert performance and explaining the cognitive processes involved. However, it would appear that there is no single 'expert way' to perform all tasks. Dorner and Scholkopf's (1991) general characterisation of expert performance is most apt, 'An expert is someone capable of doing the right thing at the right time'.

Key points Top tips

The key characteristics of an expert:

- experts are knowledgeable and have a deep level of propositional knowledge and a large volume of non-propositional knowledge
- experts are reflective practitioners
- experts are highly motivated and internally driven
- experts excel mainly in their own domain
- experts are faster at performing the skills in their domain
- experts are fast at solving problems and make few errors
- experts value the participation of relevant others in the decision-making process
- experts are patient centred
- experts share their expertise to help develop expertise in others

Rapid recap

Check your progress so far by working through each of the following questions.

1. What are the main types of leadership style?
2. What leadership styles are usually adopted by an interprofessional team leader?
3. What skills and qualities does an effective team leader possess?
4. What are the strands of professional knowledge?
5. List five of the key characteristics of an expert.

If you have difficulty with more than one of the questions, read through the section again to refresh your understanding before moving on.

References

Anderson, J.R. (1983) *The Architecture of Cognition.* Harvard University Press, Cambridge, MA.

Avolio, B.J. and Bass, B.M. (1988) Transformational leadership, charisma, and beyond. In *Emerging Leadership* (eds. Hunt, J.G., Baglia, B.R., Dachler, H.P. and Scriescheim, C.A.). Lexington Books, Lexington, MA, pp. 29–50.

Bass, B.M. (1985) *Leadership Performance Beyond Expectations.* The Free Press, New York.

Bass, B.M. and Avolio, B.J. (1994) *Improving Effectiveness through Transformational Leadership.* Thousand Oaks, Sage Publications, CA.

Boreham, N.C. (1988) Models of Diagnosis and their Implications for Adult Professional Education. In *Studies in the Education of Adults*, **20**: 95–108.

Boud, D., Cohen, R. and Walker, D. (1993) *Using Experience for Learning.* Open University Press, Milton Keynes.

Burns, J.M. (1978) *Leadership.* Harper & Row, New York.

Chi, M.T.H., Glaser, R. and Farr, M. (1988) *The Nature of Expertise.* Erlbaum, Hillsdale, NJ.

Conger, J.A. and Kanungo, R. (1988) *Charismatic Leadership: The Elusive Factor in Organisational Effectiveness.* Jossey-Bass Publishers, San Francisco, CA.

Conger, J.A. and Kanungo, R. (1998) *Charismatic Leadership in Organisations.* Thousand Oaks, Sage Publications, CA.

Department of Health (1999) *Agenda for Change: Modernising the NHS Pay System.* Department of Health, London.

Department of Health (2002) *NHS Leadership Qualities Framework.* Available from www.nhsleadershipqualities.nhs.uk.

Dorner, D. and Scholkopf, J. (1991) Controlling Complex Systems; or, Expertise as 'Grandmother's know-how'. In *Toward a General Theory of Expertise* (eds. Ericsson, K.A. and Smith, J.). Cambridge University Press, Cambridge, pp. 218–239.

Dreyfus, H.L. and Dreyfus, S.E. (1986) *Mind over Machine: The Power of Human Intuition and Expertise in the Era of the Computer.* The Free Press, New York.

Eraut, M. (1994) *Developing Professional Knowledge and Competence*. Falmer Press, London.

Ericsson, K.A. (1996) The Acquisition of Expert Performance: An Introduction to some of the Issues. In *The Road to Excellence: The Acquisition of Expert Performance in the Arts and Sciences, Sports and Games* (ed. Ericsson, K.A.). Lawrence Erlbaum Associates, USA, pp. 1–50.

Fish, D. (1998) *Appreciating Practice in the Caring Professions: Re-focusing Professional Development and Practitioner Research*. Butterworth-Heinemann, Oxford.

Glaser, R. (1984) The Role of Knowledge. *American Psychologist*, **79**(2): 93–104.

Hamm, R.M. (1999) Clinical Expertise and the Cognitive Continuum. In *Professional Judgement: A Reader in Clinical Decision Making* (eds. Dowie, J. and Elstein, A.). The Open University Press, Cambridge, pp. 78–105.

Hammond, K. (1980) *Human Judgement and Decision Making*. Hemisphere, New York.

Hersey, P. and Blanchard, K.H. (1977) *The Management of Organizational Behaviour*. Prentice Hall, Upper Saddle River, New Jersey.

Kolb, D.A. (1984) *Experiential Learning: Experience as the Source of Learning and Development*. Prentice Hall, Eaglewood Cliffs, New Jersey.

Kouzes, J.M. and Posner, B.Z. (2002) *The Leadership Challenge*. Jossey-Bass, San Diego, CA.

Minsky, M. (1977) Frame-system Theory. In *Thinking: Readings in Cognitive Science* (eds. Johnson-Laird, P.N. and Watson, P.C.). Cambridge University Press, Cambridge, pp. 355–367.

Patel, V.L., Arocha, J.F. and Kaufman, D.R. (1994) Diagnostic Reasoning and Expertise. *The Psychology of Learning and Motivation: Advances in Research Theory*. **31**: 137–252.

Patel, V.L., Arocha, J.F. and Kaufman, D.R. (1999) Expertise and Tacit Knowledge in Medicine. In *Tacit Knowledge in Professional Practice* (Sternberg, R.J. and Horvath, J.A.). Lawrence Erlbaum Associates, USA, pp. 75–99.

Patel, V.L., Kaufmann, D.R. and Magder, S.A. (1996) The Acquisition of Medical Expertise in Complex Dynamic Environments. In *The Road to Excellence: The Acquisition of Expert Performance in the Arts and Sciences, Sports and Games* (ed. Ericsson, K.A.). Lawrence Erlbaum Associates, USA, pp. 1–50.

Popper, M. and Zakkai, E. (1994) Transactional, Charismatic and Transformational Leadership: Conditions Conducive to their Predominance. *Leadership & Organisation Development Journal,* **15**(6): 3–7.

Rowden, R.W. (2000) The Relationship between Charismatic Leadership Behaviours and Organisational Commitment. In *The Leadership and Organisation Development Journal,* **21**(1): 30–35.

Ryle, G. (1949) *The Concept of Mind*. Penguin, London.

Schank, R. and Abelson, R.P. (1977) Scripts, Plans and Knowledge. In *Thinking: Readings in Cognitive Science* (eds. Johnson-Laird, P.N. and Wanson, P.C.). Cambridge University Press, Cambridge, pp. 421–432.

Schmidt, H.G., Norman, G.R. and Boshuizen, H. (1990) A Cognitive Perspective on Medical Expertise: Theory and Implications. In *Academic Medicine*, **65**(10): 611–621.

Schutz, A. (1967) *The Phenomenology of the Social World*. North Western University Press, Evanston IL.

Shamir, B., Arthur, M.B. and House, R.J. (1994) The Rhetoric of Charismatic Leadership: A Theoretical Extension, a Case Study, and Implications for Research. In *Leadership Quarterly*, **5**: 25–42.

Simon, D.P. and Simon, H.A. (1978) Individual Differences in Solving Physics Problems. In *Children's Thinking: What Develops?* (ed. Siegler, R.S.). Lawrence Erlbaum Associates, Hillsdale NJ, pp. 325–348.

Simon, H.A. and Chase, W.G. (1973) Skill in Chess. *American Scientist*, **61**: 394–403.

Stogdhill, R.M. (1974) *Handbook of Leadership: A Survey of the Literature.* Free Press, New York.

Vygotsky, L.S. (1978) *Mind in Society. The Development of Higher Psychological Processes.* Harvard University Press, Cambridge, MA.

Williams, P. (1998) Using Theories of Professional Knowledge and Reflective Practice to Influence Educational Change. *Medical Teacher*, **20**(1): 28–34.

5
Communicating with each other

Learning outcomes

By the end of this chapter you should be able to:

★ Discuss the fundamental communication skills needed to facilitate effective relationships with service users and health care professionals

★ Identify the methods of communication that enhance effective interprofessional working

★ Discuss the barriers to effective communication.

Introduction

Effective communication is considered to be essential for effective interprofessional working and the consequent delivery of quality health- and social care to patients. Communication covers a wide range of interactions including interpersonal communication, communication technology and mass communication. It also takes many forms: from brief informal conversations between professionals, to formal meetings, for example multidisciplinary team meetings; from ward rounds through to formalised written documents between professionals, for example patients records. Whether the type of communication is verbal or written the purpose is always the same, that is, the sharing of information.

All too often we have seen the tragic deaths that have occurred from a breakdown in communication within different parts of the NHS and between the NHS and other care providers such as social services. Deaths such as that of Victoria Climbié (see report, Secretary of State for Health, 2003) and the children undergoing heart surgery at Bristol Royal Infirmary (see report, Secretary of State for Health, 2001). The reports into these deaths both made recommendations related to the communication skills of health- and social-care professionals.

There can be no doubt, as these recommendations following the tragic deaths of children so vividly illustrate, about the crucial role that effective communication has in the delivery of effective patient and client care.

Prior to these tragic deaths, the government had already recognised the requirement for improved communication skills training for health professionals. The *NHS Plan* stated that:

> By 2002, it will be a pre-condition of qualification to deliver patient care in the NHS that an individual has demonstrated competence in communication with patients.
>
> Department of Health (2000)

Box 5.1

The report (Secretary of State for Health, 2001) into the deaths of children from heart surgery at Bristol Royal Infirmary

This had among its recommendations the following:

Recommendation 59

Education in communication skills must be an essential part of the education of all health care professionals. Communication skills include the ability to engage with patients on an emotional level, to listen, to assess how much information a patient wants to know and to convey information with clarity and sympathy.

Recommendation 60

Communication skills must also include the ability to engage with and respect the views of fellow health care professionals (may be there just couldn't it!).

Box 5.2

The report into the death of Victoria Climbié (Secretary of State for Health, 2003)

This had a significant number of recommendations that focused on written communication including the following:

Recommendation 12

Front-line staff in each of the agencies which regularly come into contact with families with children must ensure that with each new contact, basic information about the child is recorded. This must include the child's name, address, age, the name of the child's primary carer, the child's GP and the name of the child's school if the child is of school age.

Recommendation 38

Directors of social services must ensure that the transfer of responsibility of a case between local authority social services departments is always recorded on the case file of each authority and is confirmed in writing by the authority to which responsibility for the case has been transferred.

Recommendation 68

When concerns about deliberate harm of a child have been raised, doctors must ensure that comprehensive and contemporaneous notes are made of these concerns.

Other recommendations within the report into the death of Victoria Climbié (Secretary of State for Health, 2003) focused on the sharing and accessing of information between agencies:

Recommendation 13

The Department of Health should amalgamate the current Working Together and National Assessment Framework documents into one simplified document. The document should tackle the following six aspects in a clear and practical way:

    i) It must establish a 'common language' for use across all agencies to help those agencies to identify who they are concerned about, why they are concerned, who is best placed to respond to those concerns and what outcome is being sought from any planned response . . .

Recommendation 37

The training of social workers must equip them with the confidence to question the opinion of professionals in other agencies when conducting their own assessment of the needs of the child.

In a joint statement prepared by the Department of Health (England), Universities UK, the Health Profession's Council, the General Medical Council and the Nursing and Midwifery Council (Department of Health, 2003a) the following communication skills were identified as being necessary for students to possess at the point of registration. Students should:

- Be able to identify the communication skills required in practice to improve patient-care management and patient satisfaction with their care
- Have the ability to communicate effectively with fellow professionals and other health care staff
- Have the ability to recognise the level of their communication skills and limitations in specialist practice and be committed to personal development in these areas through post-registration and continuing professional development opportunities throughout their careers.

The deaths of Victoria Climbié and the children undergoing heart surgery at Bristol serve to further reinforce the necessity for health- and social-care professionals to possess appropriate competencies in communication skills.

We will begin this chapter by exploring the different methods of communication that are used in the health- and social-care sector to enhance interprofessional working and the quality of care delivered to patients and clients. Next, we will discuss the various types of team communication and enabling technologies. Finally, we will consider the barriers to communicating effectively within an interprofessional working environment and how these barriers might be overcome.

Methods of communication

In health- and social care, the word 'communication' covers a wide range of interactions, which can broadly be classified into two types: verbal communication and written communication.

Verbal communication

It is important to remember that, when we communicate verbally, it is not just the words and phrases of the spoken language that convey our message but also our non-verbal actions. In fact usually more information is gained from non-verbal communication than from the words that someone is actually saying. It has been found that people's attitudes and feelings are communicated 55 per cent by the body, 38 per cent by the voice and only 7 per cent by spoken words.

Being able to communicate effectively within the fields of health- and social care is paramount as it can mean the difference between life and death. A vital partnership exists between health- and social-care professionals themselves, and between health- and social-care professionals and their patients that can be either negatively or positively affected by interprofessional communication. It is, therefore, crucial that all health- and social-care professionals continuously enhance their communication skills to enable them to work effectively within an interprofessional team.

Verbal communication is the primary way in which health- and social-care professionals transmit information about a patient's care and treatment. To enhance interprofessional working, health- and social-care professionals use both formal and informal, direct (face-to-face) verbal communication strategies. Formal strategies include team meetings, ward rounds and multidisciplinary team meetings (see page 87). It has, however, been found that a large proportion of ward-based collaboration is based on informal or opportunistic interactions. These informal communication strategies include 'catching' other professionals in the hospital corridors; using care coordinators and nurses as interprofessional 'go betweens'; and verbal reports between doctors and nurses to communicate any new decisions on patient management (Reeves and Lewin, 2004, p. 224).

Verbal communication is generally much less structured and less consistent than written communication. When information is communicated verbally there are few, if any, guidelines to ensure the accuracy and completeness of the information being exchanged. There is, therefore, a risk that valuable information might be misinterpreted or lost, for example staff may forget some of the information so that an incomplete message is passed on, or staff may forget to pass the message on. If information is lost, misinterpreted or is incomplete, a breakdown of communication will result, with consequent effects on patient care. It is, therefore, essential that as health- and social-care professionals you are aware of the barriers to effective verbal communication and how these might be overcome (see page 101).

Reflective activity

Think about your practice environment and consider the following points.

- List the informal communication strategies that are used.
- What are the advantages and disadvantages of each of the strategies you have identified?
- For one of the informal communication strategies you have identified develop some guidelines and procedures to enhance the quality of the verbal communication exchanged.

Health- and social-care professionals also use indirect verbal communication which is usually used as a formal communication strategy. Indirect verbal communication is any verbal communication that is not face to face, for example via the telephone, video conferencing, teleconferencing, the answer phone.

Written communication

There are a variety of different types of written communication that health- and social-care professionals use to communicate information, including: letters, memos, fax, notice boards, e-mails, newsletters, reports, minutes from meetings, incident/accident forms. In addition to these general types of written communication, there are those that are specific to the health- and social-care setting including: prescriptions, death certificates, patient case records (see page 97); investigation request cards, medicine/drug charts, vital-signs charts.

Health- and social-care organisations have developed guidelines and procedures to address certain methods of written communication, such as which parts of the patient's case record or forms should be completed at each stage of the patient's journey to and through a team. For example, when a patient is referred for treatment, a referral form will be completed; when a patient is admitted to a ward a nursing assessment sheet will be completed; during a patient's stay in hospital a nursing care plan, vital-signs chart and a medicine/drug chart will be completed; and when a patient is discharged from the ward, a discharge plan will be completed.

Structured documents/forms designed specifically for a purpose help to ensure the type and consistency of information collected and recorded about a patient's care. They also help to ensure the completeness and accuracy of patient records.

Patient records

Patient records are a vital method of communication among professionals both within and outside of the hospital setting. Verbal dialogue between the professions often arises from the documented patient record. Patient records may be handwritten or generated using information technology. This section will consider handwritten patient records, with a later section considering electronic records. The general principles for handwritten and electronic records and record keeping are the same. Box 5.3 provides some guidelines on how good record keeping can be developed.

Box 5.3
Record keeping – good-practice guidelines

- Always ensure records are factual and accurate
- Avoid using jargon and colloquialisms
- Ensure your handwriting is legible
- Always make sure that you accurately date, time and sign the entry
- Avoid irrelevant speculation and offensive comments
- Always record information as soon as possible after the event has occurred
- Never erase any text
- Ensure that any alterations or additions are dated, timed and signed
- Only record relevant information.

NB Remember that any information you record may be scrutinised at a later date.

Adapted from guidelines for records and record keeping (NMC, 2005)

Patients' notes provide an important channel of communication as they ensure that a patient's treatment and care can be maintained if the relevant professional (for example doctor, nurse, occupational therapist, pharmacist) cannot be found on the ward or if there is insufficient time to contact them (Reeves and Lewin, 2004). Although patient records are absolutely vital for the provision of high-quality care, they should not be seen as a substitute for two-way face-to-face synchronous communication.

> ### Over to you
>
> Read the guidelines for records and record keeping that are produced by your professional body.

Patient records are covered by a number of Acts of Parliament, including the Data Protection Act 1998, the Human Rights Act 1998, Freedom of Information Act 2000 and the Access to Health Records Act 1990. All health- and social-care professionals should familiarise themselves with the salient points of each Act.

> ## Evidence base
>
> Go to the website www.dh.gov.uk/PublicationsAndStatistics/Publications/PublicationsPolicyAndGuidance/PublicationsPolicyAndGuidanceArticle/fs/en?CONTENT_ID=4131747&chk=tMmN39. Read the document Records Management: NHS Code of Practice.
>
> Go to the website www.ico.gov.uk/eventual.asp. Read the Data Protection Act 1998.

Types of meetings

Effective team communication is essential if interprofessional working is to be successful. Types of meetings that promote team communication include:

1. Team/staff meetings.
2. Multidisciplinary team meetings.
3. Ward rounds.

Team meetings

Team meetings, sometimes referred to as staff meetings, is a term used to refer to semi-formal meetings which are held in most practice environments on a regular basis. These meetings are usually chaired by the team leader/head of department/service manager.

Team meetings provide the opportunity for the team leader and team members to meet and discuss matters that affect the team. These meetings provide a two-way communication channel between the team leader and the team members and serve multiple purposes. They provide an opportunity for the team leader to share information with the team, such as issues related to the organisation in which they are working. Sharing information that affects the whole organisation and not just information related to the team makes the team members feel they are valued by the organisation and enhances their loyalty to the overall organisation and to the team.

Team meetings also enable team members to make suggestions and comments to the team leader about the ways in which the team could enhance its practice. This two-way channel of communication also enables the team leader to share with the team information that will affect the day-to-day activities of the team. If, for example, the team leader wishes to implement a change to the working practices of the team, the team meeting provides an appropriate place for this discussion to take place. All team members will be present and they can all participate in the debate and decision-making process. Commitment to any proposed changes can be increased if the team leader involves the team members in this process. Even if some of the team members do not agree with the final decision that has been made, they have had the opportunity to air their views and can understand the context within which the decision has been made.

Team meetings also bring the whole team together and although they are not primarily a social occasion, there will be opportunities for the team members to chat informally, for example before the meeting starts, during the coffee/tea break and after the meeting has finished.

The opportunity for team members to meet on a regular basis to communicate face to face with each other and the team leader is essential if the team is to function effectively. Team meetings are, however, particularly important for those teams where the professionals spend a large proportion of their time working alone, for example members of the palliative-care team or primary health care team.

Successful team meetings do not just happen and in the next section we will discuss the various steps that should be taken to increase the chances of holding an effective team meeting.

Skills required for a successful team meeting

There are a number of elements that need to be considered in order to ensure that the team meeting achieves something. These elements apply to all meetings and not just team meetings. There are three elements:

1. Preparation.
2. The meeting.
3. After the meeting.

Preparation

Preparation is the key to a successful meeting and it is the team leader who will take on this responsibility. There are a number of decisions that the team leader will have to make, including:

- **When to hold the meeting**. If the meeting is to be a regular meeting, rather than a one off, it is best if the meeting is held on the same day, at the same time and at the same frequency, for example the first Thursday of each month between 9.30 a.m. and 11.00 a.m. The frequency of this will depend on the type of meeting; for some meetings once a month may be appropriate, for others bi-monthly and for other meetings once a fortnight may be considered necessary.

  Commitment to attending a team meeting is higher if the meeting has a regular 'slot' in the calendar. This is because staff know in advance when the meeting is going to take place and can schedule other work commitments around the meeting.

- **Where to hold the meeting**. Choosing the right location for the meeting is essential. The venue should be easy for all members to reach, with adequate car-parking facilities. The room should be the right size for the number of staff expected to attend and tea/coffee-making facilities should be readily accessible. Get it wrong – venue difficult to find; no tea/coffee available; no car parking; room too small – then staff will be very reluctant to attend another meeting.

  With agreement of all the team members, it may be considered appropriate to rotate the venue of the meeting. In a primary health care team, for example, where the team may be geographically widely dispersed, rotating the venue will mean that it is not always the same members of the team travelling the longest distances. Rotating the venue, where appropriate, will increase the attendance at meetings, as no member of the team will feel that they are always being disadvantaged by having to travel a long distance.

- **Setting the agenda**. The agenda gives the meeting a structure and focus. From the agenda the team members will know why they are meeting and what they will be discussing. The purpose of the meeting, for example, might be to share information; problem solve; make decisions; or for planning and coordinating the work of the team.

  It is the team leader's responsibility to set the agenda. The agenda should be set to ensure that it keeps all team members interested and involved, while making sure that the purpose of the meeting is achieved. It is important that items for an agenda are not just generated by the team leader but that team members also contribute items. If team members have contributed to the setting of the agenda, they should feel that they have an important role in the meeting and that the team leader values their contributions to the effective functioning of the team. Box 5.4 illustrates a typical agenda.

Box 5.4

East Street palliative-care team meeting

To be held at Hawthorne House, Wednesday, 22 February 2006, 9.30 a.m. to 11.00 a.m.

AGENDA

1. Apologies for absence
2. Minutes of the previous meeting (08–02–06)
3. Matters arising
4. Proposed changes to the referral process (Paper 1 – attached)
5. Student placements within the palliative-care team (Paper 2 – attached)
6. Office space at Napier House
7. Organisation of social event for the team
8. Any other business
9. Date of next meeting.

The leader needs to give consideration to the order that items appear on the agenda. Typically, essential business items should be at the beginning of the agenda. In the specimen agenda, the crucial business item is the discussion related to the proposed changes to the referral process. The agenda should close with items that are not controversial and celebrate the success of the team. In the specimen agenda, the last topic identified for discussion is the organisation of a social event for the team. This item should ensure that the meeting closes on a high note.

The agenda and any relevant papers must be circulated to all the team members in advance of the meeting. This will enable the team members to prepare for the meeting. Team members have the responsibility to:

- on receiving the agenda and accompanying papers, check and note the day, date, time and venue for the meeting in their diary
- let the team leader know as soon as possible if they are able to attend or not. It is important that if a team member is not able to attend they send their apologies to the team leader
- ensure that prior to the meeting they have read the minutes from the previous meeting. Team members must be prepared to provide an update on any action point that they have been asked to address

- ensure that prior to the meeting they have read any relevant papers or documents so that they can contribute knowledgeably to the discussion.

The meeting

The success of a meeting will depend on how the meeting is chaired and the quality of the contributions that individual team members make during the discussions. To help facilitate successful meetings it is useful if the team agree some team ground rules. For example:

- be prepared for the meeting
- come to the meeting on time
- start and end the meeting on time
- respect and value the diversity of team members
- participate in the meeting
- actively listen to the discussions
- make decisions by consensus.

Role of the chairperson during the meeting

This is a demanding role and the success or otherwise of the meeting will depend to a large extent on whether the chair carries out their role effectively. During the meeting the chair has a number of responsibilities:

- **Opening the meeting**. It is important to start the meeting on time and with introductions if necessary. If everybody in the room does not know each other, it is important that everyone introduces themselves. It is also good practice to remind the members of the group of the purpose of the meeting and, if appropriate, housekeeping arrangements (for example, location of fire exits; toilets; tea- and coffee-making facilities) and the team ground rules. The chairperson may also ask if the team are happy with the order of the items on the agenda and changes to the order can be made at this point in the meeting if considered appropriate
- **Encouraging participation**. It is important that all group members participate in the debate. The chair will need to encourage everyone to join in; some members will need more direct encouragement than others. Using open questions, for example, 'What do you think about the proposed changes in the referral process?' is more likely to facilitate discussion than a closed question, for example, 'How much money has been spent on photocopying this month?' Closed questions are, however, useful if the chair requires specific information from the group
- **Encouraging decision making**. Making decisions is an essential part of the meeting. The chair will encourage the team to make decisions. In facilitating a decision, the chair will actively listen to

the debate, drawing together the threads of the debate and summarising the points made by the team. If appropriate, the chair will help to clarify points and ask pertinent questions of the team if there appear to be key areas of the debate that have not been explored. It is also important that the chair does not allow the team to wander off the point and that he or she ensures that if disagreements occur these are fully explored by the team before a decision is made. Decisions should be made by consensus of all the team members.

Role of the team members

A team member has the responsibility to participate in the debate and air their views on the topic being discussed. When contributing to the discussions, it is important that ideas are clearly and precisely presented. This will ensure that thoughts are effectively communicated. It is important that the team member does not become emotive about the issues that they are discussing as this will detract from the overall point that is being made. Meetings will be successful if all team members contribute, respect and value the contributions that other team members are making to the discussion, and actively listen to each other's contributions.

Role of the minute taker

It is important that minutes are taken at meetings as they form an agreed record of the discussions and decisions made at the meeting. The minutes not only record the decisions that have been made but also the action points that arise from the decision, that is, how, by whom and by when the decision is going to be implemented. At future meetings, minutes can be used to review the progress of the work of the team.

After the meeting

Even after the meeting has finished, there are a number of tasks that the chair, team members and minute taker must complete to ensure the meeting was a success.

Role of the chairperson

Following the meeting the chairperson should evaluate the meeting with the intention of improving future meetings. The following series of questions could be used as a framework for undertaking this evaluation.

- Did the meeting start and end on time?
- Was the purpose of the meeting clear?
- Did all team members contribute to the meeting?
- Did the team work toward consensus?
- Did the team identify by whom, by when and how decisions were going to be implemented?

- Was sufficient time available to debate all the issues fully?
- Was all the necessary paperwork available for the meeting?

Role of the team members

After the meeting, the team members must ensure that any action point they are responsible for is implemented within the timescale identified at the meeting.

Role of the minute taker

The minutes from a meeting should be written up as soon as possible after the meeting has finished. The final draft of the minutes should be checked for accuracy with the chair. Minutes should be circulated to all the members of the team who attended the meeting, and to those members who sent their apologies. This type of circulation list ensures that all team members are kept informed of what was achieved at the meeting.

Multidisciplinary team (MDT) meeting

There are many similarities between multidisciplinary team (MDT) meetings and team meetings. This section will therefore focus on the unique challenges of developing effective MDT meetings.

MDT membership is developed around the patient's journey through the system to ensure that all relevant professionals are able to play an active role in the care of the patient.

The following tables are three examples of MDTs and their typical membership.

Table 5.1 Head and neck cancer MDT

• Head and neck surgeon	• Specialist head and neck therapeutic radiographer
• Consultant radiologist	• MDT coordinator
• Consultant oncologist	• Clinical nurse specialist
• Macmillan radiographer	• Dentist
• Dietician	• Consultant radiologist
• Consultant histopathologist	• Speech and language therapist
• Maxillofacial surgeon	

Table 5.2 Colo-rectal cancer MDT

• Radiologist	• MDT coordinator
• Oncologist	• Nursing staff
• Histopathologist	• Diagnostic radiographer
• Specialist colo-rectal therapeutic radiographer	• Surgeon
• Research and development nurses	

Table 5.3 shows an MDT that has been set up in two primary schools in the Borough of Camden. The purpose of these two MDTs is to enable agencies to work together more effectively to improve outcomes for children. The MDT consists of school staff and other professionals from outside the schools who already provide a service to the school. This is an excellent example of interprofessional working across three sectors: health, social services and education.

Table 5.3 Camden Children's Fund MDT (The Department for Education and Skills, 2006)

• Head teacher • Home school liaison worker	• Child protection designated teacher • Education support officer for a community scheme for African/ Caribbean children
• Administrator	• Manager, Camden primary schools project
• Specialist teachers from the learning support services • Special educational needs coordinator • Child and adolescent psychotherapist • Learning mentor • Education welfare officer	• Speech and language therapist • Social worker • School nurse • Educational psychologist • Paediatric occupational therapist

As these three examples illustrate, the number of different professionals involved in one MDT can be in excess of 10 people and this provides unique challenges for developing effective MDT meetings.

What are the challenges for MDT meetings?

The challenges for developing effective communication channels for an MDT meeting can be divided into three broad areas:

1. Coordinating the MDT meeting.
2. Time commitment.
3. Resources.

Coordinating the MDT meeting

MDTs will normally have an MDT coordinator who will provide administrative/secretarial support before, during and after the MDT meeting. The MDT coordinator is crucial to the smooth running of the MDT meeting and to streamlining the patient pathway. The key responsibilities of the coordinator include:

• arranging the meeting
• obtaining the list of patients to be discussed at the meeting

- getting the patient's details, for example patients notes, imaging, histopathology reports
- recording attendance at the meetings
- recording decisions made about a patient's/client's treatment and management on the MDT pro forma
- booking and tracking appointments and tests for patients
- ensuring effective communication between the MDT and its related teams in primary, secondary and tertiary care.

The MDT coordinator is therefore at the hub of the MDT and is of crucial importance to effective communications between core members of the MDT, members of the extended MDT and the patient. The MDT coordinator must possess excellent verbal and written communication skills which can be adapted and applied to the broad-ranging situations they will meet.

Time commitment

The majority of MDTs meet on a weekly basis and meetings are usually scheduled for 60–90 minutes. Core members or their agreed cover are expected to attend the majority of meetings. Although the actual MDT meeting may only last for 90 minutes, members need time to make sure that all the relevant images have been reviewed in advance of the meeting. Time is also required after the meeting to carry out any tasks resulting from decisions taken at the MDT meeting. As people may be members of many MDTs, the time commitment for individuals will not be insignificant.

Resources

To facilitate the effective functioning of an MDT meeting, specific resources are made available. The meeting room will have image-viewing equipment and equipment for viewing pathology slides. This means that all members of the MDT can view the patient information at the same time, allowing each member to make their own unique contribution to the discussion about the patient's treatment and management plan.

Another resource that can aid the communication process at an MDT meeting is the availability of a laptop computer with projection facilities. This facility enables the MDT coordinator to type decisions made directly onto the MDT pro forma, which can then be viewed and agreed by those members present. At end of the MDT meeting, therefore, all the decisions made have been electronically recorded and agreed as accurate. The decisions from the MDT meeting can then be communicated electronically to all relevant parties, for example members of the MDT, the patient's GP, palliative-care team, within 24 hours.

Video conferencing facilities are another resource that can aid communication between members of the MDT. This resource is invaluable as it allows for cross-site communication, allowing core members from different sites to participate in the MDT meeting without needing to spend time on travelling.

As can be seen, an MDT meeting may use the entire range of communication methods: face to face, telephone, written, e-mail, video conferencing and IT equipment, to enhance the effective working of the MDT. This should result in the patient receiving the most suitable care from diagnosis through treatment to follow-up care and support with the least delay. This will contribute to improved patient outcome.

Health professional speaks

Morag, a senior mammographer, discusses her perceptions of the breast multi-disciplinary meetings that she attends:

A meeting of minds who come together to make decisions regarding the future of a patient's care. That is my view of an MDT meeting and in my experience this is the end result. All members of the team are looking at the x-ray films and the pathology. This is done with the chairperson reciting the clinical history from the notes. When all the information has been examined then a discussion ensues as to the next step.

The stronger members of the team, surgeons and oncologists can have a difference of opinion. Which is quite amusing to the rest of us. The pathologists can use the venue to pass opinion as to what surgery still needs to be done.

The meeting can be a very uplifting experience, successful treatment followed by breast-conserving surgery and a good prognosis will give a good feeling about the worthiness of it all. Alternatively patient following patient, all young with advanced disease can be very disheartening.

On the whole a good MDT meeting will allow all in attendance to have a voice, as each profession when they meet the patient will have picked up on different aspects of her needs and by sharing this information the patient experience can only be enhanced.

Over to you

Go to the website www.ebc-indevelopment.co.uk/mdt/intro.htm . On this website, the Cancer Services Collaborative Improvement Partnership has provided a useful Multidisciplinary Team Resource guide. Read this guide to help you understand MDTs and MDT meetings.

Ward rounds

A ward round is a daily meeting organised by the ward to discuss and plan with the patient their short- and long-term care needs. The patient, their relatives and/or significant others, the medical team and a member of the nursing team will normally be present during the ward round. Other professionals may also participate in the ward round if they are involved in planning the patient's care. For example, on a stroke rehabilitation ward, a physiotherapist, an occupational therapist and a speech and language therapist may also be present.

Following the two-way face-to-face communications which take place during the ward round, the discussions and decisions made about a patient's care and treatment must be documented in writing in the patient's case records (see page 98).

In some hospitals, modern technology is being used to enhance the efficiency of ward rounds. 'Mobile carts', which are personal computers on wheels, are being used to enable doctors, nurses and other relevant staff to perform various tasks at the patient's bedside which previously had to be undertaken at a shared personal computer at the ward reception desk. The mobile cart is wirelessly connected to the hospital computer network.

The mobile cart can be used for ordering prescriptions, finding test results and, crucially, recording the discussions and decisions made by the ward-round team at the patient's bedside. Recording information in real time improves the accuracy in recording information, and being able to order prescriptions and investigations immediately means that the patient's treatment pathway is smoother and more expedient (NHS Wales Informing Health care, 2006).

Ward rounds have the added benefit of providing an interprofessional learning opportunity by emphasising the different perspectives and contributions made to patient care by the different team members.

Students speaking

Joelle, a third-year adult nursing student, talks of her experiences of attending ward rounds.

I have been fortunate to have been involved in many interprofessional ward rounds, and been actively encouraged by my mentors to accompany the other members of the team. This has helped me understand how the management of patient care is organised, while also gaining a greater understanding of the role of various members of the multiprofessional team.

However, there have also been times when I have been aware of the boundaries that still exist between some health care professionals and how stepping out of these boundaries and working collectively is difficult for some.

Enabling technologies

Traditionally, the transfer of information between health care professionals, patients and other agencies has relied upon letters or telephone calls and much of the transfer has relied on information carried by patients (Department of Health, 2005). In the 21st century, the new information technologies are being used and developed to enable information to be shared effectively between teams and organisations.

In April 2005, NHS Connecting for Health, an agency of the Department of Health, was launched. Its primary role is to deliver new, integrated IT systems and services to help modernise the NHS and ensure that care is centred around the patient. The new IT systems and services which are being delivered by NHS Connecting for Health are:

- NHS care records service
- Choose and book service
- Electronic transmission of prescriptions
- National network
- Contact
- Picture archiving and communications systems (PACS)
- IT supporting GPs.

Department of Health (2005)

In this section, we will discuss two of these new IT systems and services, electronic records and PACS, and consider how these technologies will enhance interprofessional working.

Electronic records

Patient records are the key to the delivery of high-quality health and social care. There are numerous government documents and reports that highlight the necessity for single interprofessional patient records that can be accessed by the patient and all those professionals caring for them. These documents include *Essence for Care* (Department of Health, 2003b), the *National Service Framework for Older People* (Department of Health, 2001) and the *Victoria Climbié Enquiry* (Secretary of State for Health, 2003). Electronic records have facilitated the implementation of interprofessional single-patient records. There are two types of electronic record:

- **Electronic patient record (EPR)** – this is a record of the periodic care a patient receives from a particular institution. The EPR is, therefore, all the patient's notes in an electronic format (Department of Health, 1998).
- **Electronic health record (EHR)** – this is a longitudinal record, held in primary care that contains a note of any contact with health services during the life of the patient. It includes both primary-care information and subsets of the EPR (Department of Health, 1998).

It is intended that, by 2008, patients will be able to electronically access their electronic health record via a secure web service called Healthspace (Department of Health, 2006). The Healthspace website has already been launched and over the next few years the site will be expanded to give patients more choice and control over their own health and care.

Electronic records accentuate the need for a common method for communicating patient information. Currently different professions use different documentation systems, which means that there is variation in the detail of information that is recorded, potentially leading to less than optimal patient care. In an attempt to standardise the structure and type of information collected, the NHS Headings Project (NHS Information Authority, 2003) has developed and evaluated a semi-structured pro forma. The pro forma consists of two sections:

- **Health characteristics** – this section documents the state of the patient and was organised under seven headings: history, family history, social circumstances, examination findings, test results, diagnosis and outcome.

- **Actions** – this section documents anything that can be done to or for a patient in the process of health care. Actions are organised under four headings: assessment, treatment, clinical administration and participation.

A standard, semi-structured approach to recording patient information offers health care professionals a system of communication that provides consistency of content, but also, importantly, provides the opportunity to record the detail of the consultation with the patient, ensuring that no information is lost.

Evidence base

The NHS Headings Project website provides further detail on the interprofessional patient documentation system.
Go to website: www.nhsia.nhs.uk/headings/pages/draftinfo.asp.

It is important that health- and social-care professionals are aware of the legal aspects of working with electronic records. All the Acts of Parliament that apply to manual records also apply to electronic records. These are the Data Protection Act 1998; the Access to Health Records Act 1990 and the Freedom of Information Act 2000. There are, however, additional considerations that need to be given to the management of electronic records, which include the use, storage, security and retrieval of records and compliance with the Computer Misuse Act 1990. All health- and social-care professionals should familiarise themselves with these additional requirements for the handling of electronic records.

Evidence base

Go to website www.open.gov.uk/doh/coinh.htm and read the document
'HSC1998/153 Using Electronic Patient Records in Hospitals: Legal Requirements
and Good Practice'.

Go to website www.hmso.gov.uk and familiarise yourself with the Computer
Misuse Act 1990.

Go to website www.csp.org.uk and read the document 'General Principles of
Record Keeping and Access to Health Records'. This document has been
produced by the Chartered Society of Physiotherapy and provides some useful
information for all health professionals on the management of electronic records.

There can be no doubt that the introduction of electronic single-patient/
health records will enhance communication across an interprofessional
team. Electronic records are easier to read, less bulky and reduce the
need for professionals to re-record information that has already been
recorded by another professional. A good example of information that is
duplicated if profession-specific records are maintained is the patient's
medical history. How often do we ask a patient a question about
their medical history to be asked, 'Don't you all talk to each other? I told
the nurse/doctor/physiotherapist that.'

Electronic records will be invaluable to all interprofessional teams,
but particularly for those teams that are geographically dispersed, for
example primary-care teams.

Picture archiving and communication systems (PACS)

PACS is a system which captures, stores, distributes and displays static
or moving digital images such as radiographs, CT, ultrasound, MR,
nuclear medicine. The system takes away any need to print on film and
to file or distribute images manually. It is planned that PACS will be
enabled across the NHS in England by 2007 (Department of Health,
2005).

The benefits of PACS for effective interprofessional working and the
consequent enhancement of patient care are several. As PACS stores
images digitally, it means that the images can be distributed to any
number of workstations simultaneously. This allows team members to
view the same information across one or more locations at the same
time, enabling more discussion and collaborative working to the benefit
of the patient.

PACS are ideal for use during multidisciplinary team meetings
(MDTs). As each patient is discussed, the relevant images can be
retrieved and displayed so that the entire MDT can view them at the
same time. Without PACS, the images would need to be displayed on a
light box, which means that the images are not of sufficient size for the

whole team to view simultaneously. As a result, the use of PACs means that the discussion and decisions about a patient's treatment and care plan are fully informed by information provided by the images. As PACS is a central database, it also means that if a patient has had images taken at a different NHS Trust to where they are currently being treated, the images can also be retrieved instantaneously. There is no longer the need to wait for images to arrive from another hospital or to rely on patients carrying packets of film around the hospital and between sites during the course of their care.

PACS also enables clinicians to access specialist opinion from anywhere within the NHS across England, that is, the acute, primary-care and community settings. The benefits to the patient are evident, no longer does the patient have to be living in a particular part of England to have specialist input into their treatment and care plan. For the professionals involved in the discussions with the specialist, it provides an interprofessional learning opportunity.

It is clear to see that PACS has the potential to enhance interprofessional learning and interprofessional working between health care professionals. For the patient, their experience of the care they receive will be considerably enhanced, culminating in improved care planning and possibly quicker discharge from hospital.

Over to you

Go to the website www.connectingforhealth.nhs.uk. Read about the following IT systems and services being developed and implemented by NHS Connecting for Health:

- Electronic transmission of prescriptions
- Contact.

For each service consider how it will enhance interprofessional collaboration.

What are the barriers to interprofessional communication?

In the previous sections we have considered verbal and written methods of communication and enabling technologies as ways in which interprofessional communication and therefore interprofessional working can be enhanced. However, the effectiveness of these communication methods and technologies depends entirely on the communication skills of the individual professional and the context within which they are working. The communication process is illustrated in Figure 5.1.

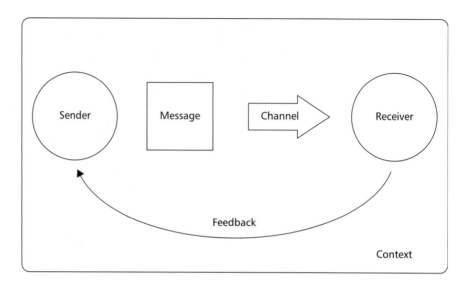

Figure 5.1 The communication process (taken from http://www.mindtools.com/ CommSkill/CommunicationIntro.htm and used with permission.)

Barriers to communication can occur at any stage of the communication process and have the potential to create misunderstandings and confusion. As a health- and social-care professional, it is important that you have an awareness of the possible barriers to communication and at what point these may occur in the communication process. This will enable you to take the appropriate steps to break down the barriers and deliver your information effectively.

There are many potential barriers to communication including:

- **Inappropriate channel of communication selected** – for example, selecting a written method when face-to-face communication would have been better or vice versa.
- **Distractions** – for example, other people talking, equipment, noise, televisions, radios, interruptions.
- **Hierarchy** – the hierarchal nature of health care creates power gaps that contribute to less than optimal communication between different professionals and with patients (see Chapter 7).
- **Lack of time** – to communicate effectively takes time, and the pressures of the workplace may result in the health care professionals doing another task or thinking about what they are going to do next at the same time as a message is being communicated to them. As a consequence, the health care professional is not fully concentrating and focusing on the person speaking and this may result in vital information being lost or misinterpreted.

- **Complex messages** – communication within and between professionals is often complex and as a result frequently lengthy. A complex lengthy message will increase the chances of the message being misunderstood or misinterpreted.

- **Ideological differences between health care professions** – different professional groups have different viewpoints according to their professional role. While this may be viewed positively, as each professional is able to contribute their expertise to the care of the patient, it can also present challenges to effective interprofessional communication. Different viewpoints arising from ideological differences can make effective communication more difficult (see Chapter 7).

- **Too much information** – this may result in information overload. If too much information is provided it is difficult for the person receiving the information to extract the salient points. It is best to be precise and only include relevant information, as this will increase the likelihood that the message will be effectively communicated. Often less really is more.

- **Professional language** – different professional groups use different professional language, which can lead to problems of understanding each other (see Chapter 7).

- **Professional jargon** – professionals frequently use jargon when communicating with patients. This is likely to result in the patient receiving incomplete information because they are unable to understand all the information being communicated by the professional.

- **Too many communications** – in busy and complex environments, such as those found in health care, a health care professional will receive numerous communications on a daily basis. These communications may be via the telephone or e-mail or during a ward round or team meeting. With so many communications, it can be difficult, if not impossible, to determine which communications are most critical.

Case study

Exploring barriers to effective communication

You are at the nurses' station on the ward completing paperwork. A relative of one of your patients comes to the nurses' station and is clearly anxious about their relative. They wish to discuss the care of their relative with you. The telephone rings and you are the only member of staff around.

With reference to the case study:

- What are the barriers to communication that exist in this scenario?
- How could you overcome these barriers?
- How would you deal with this situation?

Key points | Top tips

The potential barriers to communication are:

- distractions
- hierarchy
- inappropriate channel of communication
- too many communications
- complex messages
- professional language
- too much information
- ideological differences between different professionals
- lack of time

RRRRR**Rapid recap**

Check your progress so far by working through each of the following questions.

1. What are the main methods of verbal communication?
2. What are the benefits of multidisciplinary team meetings?
3. How do electronic single-patient/health records enhance interprofessional communication?
4. What factors inhibit interprofessional communication?

If you have difficulty with more than one of the questions, read through the section again to refresh your understanding before moving on.

References

Carr, J. and Sheikh, A. (2003) Telephone Consultations. *BMJ*, **326**: 966–969.

Carr, J. and Sheikh, A. (2004) Email Consultations in Health Care: 1 Scope and Effectiveness. *BMJ*, **329**: 435–438.

Carr, J. and Sheikh, A. (2004) Email Consultations in Health Care: 2 Acceptability and Safe Application. *BMJ*, **329**: 439–442.

Department for Education and Skills (2006) *Camden Children's Fund MDT.* Available from: www.everychildmatters.gov.uk.

Department of Health (1998) *Information for Health: An Information Strategy for the Modern NHS 1998–2005.* NHSE, London.

Department of Health (2000) *The NHS Plan: A Plan for Investment, a Plan for Reform.* HMSO, London. Available from: www.dh.gov.uk.

Department of Health (2001) *National Service Framework for Older People.* HMSO, London. Available from: www.dh.gov.uk.

Department of Health (2003a) *Guiding Principles Relating to the Commissioning and Provision of Communication.* Department of Health, Leeds. Available from: www.dh.gov.uk.

Department of Health. (2003b) *Essence of Care: Patient-focused Benchmarking for Health Care Practitioners.* HMSO, London. Available from: www.dh.gov.uk.

Department of Health (2005) *Connecting for Health.* Available from: www.connecting forhealth.nhs.uk/.

Department of Health (2006) *NHS Healthspace* (2006) Available from: www.nhs.uk/ healthspace.

NHS Information Authority (2003) *NHS Heading Project.* Available from: www.nhsia.nhs.uk/headings/pages/default.asp.

NHS Wales Informing Health care (2006) *A New Dimension to Ward Rounds.* Available from: www.wales.nhs.uk/ihc/news.cfm?contentid=3412.

Nursing and Midwifery Council. (2005) *Guidelines for Records and Record Keeping.* London: NMC. Available from: www.nmc-uk.org.

Reeves, S. and Lewin, S. (2004) Interprofessional Collaboration in the Hospital: Strategies and Meaning. *Journal of Health Services Research & Policy,* **9**(4): 218–226.

Secretary of State for Health (2001) *Learning from Bristol.* The Stationery Office, London.

Secretary of State for Health (2003) *The Victoria Climbié Inquiry.* The Stationery Office, London.

The Chartered Society of Physiotherapy (2000) *General Principles of Record Keeping and Access to Health Records.* The Chartered Society of Physiotherapy, London. Available from: www.csp.org.uk.

6
Interprofessional learning within a practice environment

Learning outcomes

By the end of this chapter you should be able to:

★ Discuss the developments in interprofessional learning

★ Understand situated learning theory

★ Create a learning environment within which effective interprofessional learning can take place

★ Critically appraise the concept of interprofessional mentorship.

Introduction

The tragic deaths of young children such as Maria Colwell (Department of Health and Social Security, 1974), the children undergoing heart surgery at Bristol Royal Infirmary (Secretary of State for Health, 2001) and Victoria Climbié (Secretary of State for Health, 2003) indicate that despite all of the rhetoric, health- and social-care professionals, whether working in the statutory, voluntary or private sectors are still not effectively collaborating. The reports into these deaths have suggested both implicitly and explicitly that 'shared learning' is one of the key methods by which collaboration could be cultivated and encouraged.

There can be no doubt, as the reports into these tragic deaths so vividly illustrate, that effective interprofessional collaboration between health- and social-care professionals will enhance the patient outcome. It is not only in cases of child abuse investigation that the significance of interprofessional collaboration can be seen on patient outcomes. Examples of enhanced patient outcomes through collaboration can be found in a range of settings, for example primary care and acute care and rehabilitation. But is 'interprofessional learning' the panacea that we have been searching for to facilitate effective interprofessional working? The fundamental questions that need to be addressed are:

● Does interprofessional education actually enhance interprofessional working?

● Does interprofessional education actually enhance patient outcomes?

As yet, we do not know the answer to these questions. A large-scale systematic review undertaken by Zwarenstein *et al.* (2001) to assess the usefulness of interprofessional education interventions found that, despite the large body of literature, the studies lacked the methodological rigour needed to convincingly understand the impact of interprofessional education on professional practice and/or health care outcomes.

We will begin this chapter by discussing the UK health- and social-care policies that have influenced the developments of interprofessional learning. Next, we will examine the concept of situated learning and the creation of a 'situated learning environment' within which effective interprofessional learning can be engendered. Finally we will consider the importance of supporting learners within the practice environment. Mentorship and in particular interprofessional mentorship and how this role might be developed in the future will be explored, with reference to professional, statutory and regulatory requirements.

What are the drivers for interprofessional learning?

The drivers for interprofessional learning mirror those for interprofessional working:

1. The changing health- and social-care environment
2. New government policies and initiatives
3. High-profile child-abuse cases
4. Professional developments
5. Technological developments.

In Chapter 2 we discussed these drivers with particular reference to interprofessional working. In this section we will focus on the UK health- and social-care policies and initiatives that have influenced the development of interprofessional learning and, where appropriate, we will refer to the other drivers.

The findings of public inquiries into the deaths of children have significantly influenced the developments in the education and training of all health- and social-care professionals.

Boxes 6.1 and 6.2 detail the recommendations following from two of the most high-profile cases.

As can be seen from the recommendations, both inquiries identified the need to radically reform the education and training of a range of professionals to promote collaborative working focused on the patient. The Department of Health responded to these recommendations with the publication of a number of White Papers. These White Papers outlined proposed changes to the way in which health- and social-care professionals would be educated in the future.

Making a Difference: Strengthening the Nursing, Midwifery and Health Visiting Contribution to Health and Health care (Department of Health, 1999)

In this White Paper, the government outlined proposals to modernise education, training and regulation in nursing, midwifery and health visiting. This included providing more flexible career pathways into and within nursing; increasing the level of practical skills within the training

Box 6.1

Learning from Bristol (Secretary of State for Health, 2001)

This report into children's heart surgery at Bristol Royal Infirmary had among its 200 recommendations the following:

Recommendation 57

Greater priority than at present should be given to non-clinical aspects of care in six key areas in the education, training and continuing professional development of health care professionals:

- Skills in communicating with patients and with colleagues
- Education about the principles and organisation of the NHS and about how care is managed, and the skills required for management
- The development of teamwork
- Shared learning across professional boundaries
- Clinical audit and reflective practice
- Leadership.

Recommendation 61

The education, training and continuing professional development (CPD) of all health care professionals should include joint courses between the professions.

Recommendation 62

There should be more opportunities than at present for multiprofessional teams to learn, train and develop together.

Box 6.2

Victoria Climbié Report (Secretary of State for Health, 2003)

Similarly the report into the death of Victoria Climbié had among its recommendations the following:

Recommendation 14

Each of the training bodies covering services provided by doctors, nurses, teachers, police officers, officers working in housing departments and social workers to demonstrate that effective joint working between each of these professional groups features in their national programmes.

Although the inquiries into the death of Victoria Climbié and the deaths of children undergoing heart surgery at the Bristol Royal Infirmary were set up in response to very different service failures, both reports had a consistent theme; the extent to which traditional divisions and demarcations between professions appeared to impede the need to work collaboratively in the interests of the patient.

programmes and delivering a nurse training system that was more responsive to the needs of the NHS. In the provision of continuing professional development (CPD), NHS organisations were to ensure that education programmes were focused on the development needs of clinical teams across traditional professional and service boundaries.

The NHS Plan – A Plan for Investment, a Plan for Reform (Department of Health, 2000a)

In this White Paper there was a clear commitment to providing pre-registration interprofessional education programmes for health- and social-care professionals. The White Paper stated:

> There will be new joint training across professions in communication skills and in NHS principles and organisation. They will form part of a new care curriculum for all education programmes for NHS staff. By 2002 it will be a pre-condition of qualification to deliver patient care in the NHS that an individual has demonstrated competence in communication with patients. A new common foundation programme will be put into place to enable students and staff to switch careers and training paths more easily.
>
> Department of Health (2000a)

Meeting the Challenge: A Strategy for the Allied Health Professions (Department of Health, 2000b)

This White Paper outlined how education, training and regulation were to be modernised within the allied health professions and was based on the same general principles for modernising the education, training and regulation for nurses, midwives and health visitors (Department of Health, 1999). Proposals outlined in this White Paper included more:

- flexible pathways into and through pre-registration programmes with opportunities to step on and off
- part-time programmes
- opportunities for shared learning
- innovative approaches to practice and fieldwork placements.

A Health Service of all the Talents: Developing the NHS Workforce (Department of Health, 2000c)

In this White Paper, the government again confirmed its commitment to develop education and training arrangements which were 'genuinely' multiprofessional and which would enable students to transfer easily between courses without having to start their training from the beginning again.

Working Together, Learning Together: A Framework for Lifelong Learning for the NHS (Department of Health, 2001)

This White Paper stated that all universities in England offering pre-registration professional education programmes should include common learning by 2004. Part of the government's commitment to the implementation of common learning was the funding of four 'leading-edge' sites. In 2002, the four leading-edge sites were announced. They were the higher education institutions at Newcastle; Kings College, London; Sheffield Hallam; and Southampton (Department of Health, 2002). These leading-edge sites had a broad remit which included to:

- develop common-learning programmes and core curricula for all professional staff in communications and NHS principles
- change workforce practices
- develop new ways of working
- break down professional and organisational barriers to learning and working together through closer integration of health professional programmes.

Evidence base

The following websites provide information on the common-learning projects that have been developed, implemented and evaluated by each of the four leading-edge sites. These websites are a very good resource for information on interprofessional learning.

- Sheffield Hallum University www.cuilu.group.shef.ac.uk/
- Southampton University www.hciu.soton.ac.uk/2_innovations/1_projects/commonlearning
- University of Newcastle www.ncl.ac.uk/teachingexcellence/researchled/projects/common/htm
- Kings College, London www.kcl.ac.uk/ipe/intro/index.html.

As can be seen, since 1999 when the White Paper *Making a Difference* (Department of Health, 1999) was published, there have been four significant White Papers which have shaped the education and training of health- and social-care professionals as we have moved into the 21st century. In this section, only key health- and social-care education and training policies have been discussed. There have, however, been other policies published which relate to specific service provision, for example child health (Department for Education and Skills, 2005) and specific professions, for example social work (University of Salford, 2004).

What is situated learning?

This exploration of situated learning will be based on the work of Lave (1988) and Lave and Wenger (1991). Lave and Wenger (1991) are key proponents in the field of situated learning.

Lave and Wenger's (1991) theory of situated learning evolved from the historical forms of apprenticeship, whereby students spent a considerable period of time, usually five years, learning their craft from a 'master'. This form of training focuses on the gradual acquisition of craft knowledge through demonstration and practice, with feedback. Until recently, learning through apprenticeship was assumed to be concrete, context-embedded, intuitive, limited in scope of its application, mechanical, rote, imitative, not creative, and out of date. However, recently there has been renewed interest in situated learning as a model of how professionals learn to apply practical knowledge within infinitely varied social contexts. Central to Lave and Wenger's (1991) theory is a process called 'legitimate peripheral participation'. This is a rather complex term and can be best understood by considering the three components of this phrase separately. All three components depend on each other:

1. It is **legitimate** because everyone involved accepts the position of learners/new team members/newly qualified practitioners as potential members of the community of practice.

2. **Peripheral** because the 'potential' members of the community of practice are initially observing practice from the periphery on the edge, before gradually becoming more and more involved with the practices of the community.

3. **Participation** because it is through 'doing' that they acquire knowledge. Knowledge is situated within the community of practice, rather than something that exists in textbooks.

Lave and Wenger (1991) claimed that this process provided a means for understanding how apprentices' understanding and knowledgeable skills develop in practice. Initially newcomers' 'legitimate peripherality' involves participation as a way of learning the 'culture of practice' and the opportunity to make the culture theirs. Thus, from a largely peripheral perspective, apprentices gradually gain a general idea of what constitutes the practice of the community. Over a period of time, the newcomers' understanding of old-timers increases, for example newcomers know how, when and about what old-timers collaborate, disagree/agree about and what they enjoy, dislike, respect and admire. The process of 'legitimate peripheral participation' provides the newcomers with exemplars as they move towards full participation in the community of practice. Partial participation is a dynamic process in which the newcomer can gain access to sources of understanding through growing involvement in the community of practice.

Lave and Wenger's (1991) theory moves the focus of learning away from the individual towards the community, emphasising the view that learning is an integral and inseparable aspect of social practice.

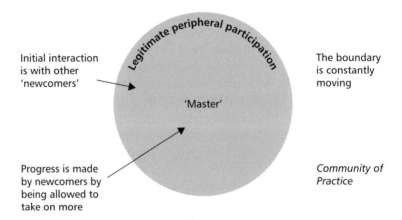

Initial interaction is with other 'newcomers'

Legitimate peripheral participation

'Master'

The boundary is constantly moving

Progress is made by newcomers by being allowed to take on more

Community of Practice

Figure 6.1 Diagram to illustrate 'legitimate peripheral participation'

NB The diagram is not endorsed by Lave and Wenger (1991) and is purely representational

The key features of a community of practice are:

- Communities of practice are everywhere – at home, at work, at university. We all belong to a number of them.
- Communities of practice are informally bound by what they do together and by what they have learned through their mutual engagement in these activities.
- Communities of practice develop around things that matter to people.
- The practices of a community reflect the members' own understanding of what is important.
- Communities of practice are defined by what the community is about; how it functions and what capability it has produced.

Reflective activity

Think of a community of practice that you have been involved in as a 'newcomer' and consider the following:

- Who was involved in the community of practice?
- Draw a diagram to show who you interacted with and who interacted with you.
- Who did you respect and why?
- What did the old-timers enjoy about working within the community of practice?
- What did the old-timers debate/discuss/disagree with each other about?
- Think about how well the community of practice functioned as a team.

What are the criticisms of situated learning theory?

We will now consider some of the criticisms that have been levied at the situated learning theory. 'Legitimate peripheral participation' has been criticised as an approach to learning as it is difficult to see how communities of practice can be critiqued and changed. There is a real possibility that practices could stagnate in communities where there are no new ideas being introduced. If no new ideas are being injected into the practice setting, the knowledge and skills of practitioners will not be advanced and eventually the quality of care provided to the patient will be adversely affected. But people in these communities do, of course, have to find a way to adapt to influences for change that come from beyond the community itself. Shotter raises our awareness of the problems that can result from a stagnate practice setting:

> The members of an institution need not necessarily have been its originators, they may be second, third, fourth etc. generation members, having inherited the institution from their forebears . . . This is a most important point, for although there may be an intentional structure to institutional activities, practitioners of institutional forms need have no awareness at all of the reasons for its structure – for them it is just 'the way things are done'. The reasons for the institution having one form rather than another is buried in its history.
>
> Shotter (cited in Rogoff, 1990, p. 45)

 Case study

A community of practice in action

Alan is a junior therapeutic radiographer and is concerned about the reluctance of senior professionals to change practices within his community. He feels that the radiotherapy techniques are 'set in stone' and that because the senior radiographers have always done it that way, then that is the way it will always be. The more senior members of staff have trained and practised within the same community and, therefore, have no experience of practices in other communities. In addition, many of the older consultants have been at this hospital for 30–40 years and just tend to do what they have always done. Alan knows that practices could be enhanced, and does make suggestions, but the suggestions are always ignored by the senior staff and the older consultants.

1. What are the implications for Alan's community of practice if the old-timers continue to oppose making changes to practice?

2. Why do the old-timers feel unable to collaborate with Alan as a newcomer?

3. What do you feel could be done to create an environment in which the old-timers and newcomers could learn together to continuously develop new knowledge and skills?

Lave and Wenger (1991), however, believe that, because the focus is on the community of practice and not the individual, the development of the community depends on the positions that newcomers can or cannot find within the community of practice and the relationships that can or cannot be set up between the newcomers and the political, economical and cultural life of the community.

All the individuals within a community of practice have different interests and make different contributions to the activities of that community and hold different viewpoints. Therefore, the organisation of the community, 'its power relations and its conditions for legitimacy define the possibilities for learning' (Lave and Wenger, 1991, p. 98). The community of practice will not stagnate because the focus for learning has moved from the master-apprentice relationship to the organisation of the community of practice of which the master is a part. Thus, in a community of practice, understanding and knowledge is created as individuals become involved in the various activities of the community and interact with different people over a period of time.

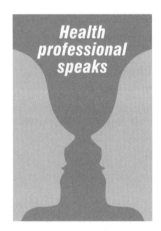

Health professional speaks

Keiko, a qualified Operating Department Practitioner, talks about her work environment also being a learning environment.

With my colleagues we do tend to swap articles, if you've got some good articles. For example, I recently studied on the Preparation for Mentorship module, and a couple of my colleagues had already completed this course and they had some really relevant articles and they bought them in and shared them with me. Or you might come across a good reference related to anaesthetics or they give it to you and you are then able to look it up, so yes, we do share tips, our knowledge, to improve our professional knowledge and enhance our patient care.

Another criticism made of the situated learning theory is that it does not see a role for reflecting on practice. As we know, the process of reflection is a key aspect of professional learning at all stages of our professional career. Therefore, it is of concern if situated learning theory does not advocate reflection. So what do Lave and Wenger (1991) say about reflection? In fact, although they do not explicitly mention reflection, Lave and Wenger (1991, p. 108) do acknowledge the important role that reflection plays in the development of a community of practice, making a distinction between talking about and talking within a practice:

> Talking within itself includes both talking within (e.g. exchanging information necessary to the progress of ongoing activities) and talking about (e.g. stories, community lore). Inside the shared practice both forms of talk fulfil specific

functions: engaging, focusing, and shifting attention bringing about co-ordination, etc., on the one hand, and supporting communal forms of memory and reflection, as well as signalling membership, on the other.

Lave and Wenger (1991, p. 108)

From this quotation, Lave and Wenger appear to be seeing the community of practice as a place where professionals use their professional judgement to make decisions while they are practising. This activity is very similar to that of a professional reflecting-in-practice (Schon, 1983).

Key points | Top tips

- Situated learning theory recognises that knowledge is embedded within the context in which it is used and cannot be separated from the activity, context and culture of that situation
- Learners engage in situated learning by negotiating meaning with one another through the use of tools and artefacts such as language, books, music and art
- Learning takes place as a result of participating in 'real' activities that nurture and guide the learner's ability to think
- Learners develop a shared understanding about the purpose of the community and develop a sense of belonging

---

How to create an interprofessional situated-learning environment

We will now consider the specific approaches toward learning and teaching which a community of practice could embrace to create an interprofessional situated-learning environment. These features centre on fostering varied learning and teaching strategies that encourage the newcomers and old-timers of a community of practice to develop both personally and professionally. These learning and teaching strategies include frameworks for learning (for example critical appreciation, cooperative learning, collaboration, coaching) and tools for learning (for example reflection, narratives). We will discuss these frameworks and tools below.

Frameworks for learning

Critical appreciation

Critical appreciation, a term that comes from the arts, is a process to enable practitioners to express their insights into professional practice.

It is concerned with recognising, in a sensitive and holistic way, the qualities of practice and thinking critically about the values, traditions, beliefs and assumptions that underlie its surface (Fish, 1989). It involves the practitioners themselves investigating their own work but as part of their normal duties. A key activity in critical appreciation is for practitioners to bring the personal professional knowledge embedded in their practice to the surface and to consider it critically in the light of the context, the traditions and conventions of their profession as a whole.

Critical appreciation is not unproblematic, because for many health- and social-care professions, particularly scientific-based professions, the idea of conceptualising practice as art and seeing their work as artistry is an alien concept. Therefore, initially, a great deal of time would need to be invested by the members of a community to help both newcomers and old-timers to develop the skills and language that are necessary for artistic writing. Also, the success of professional artistry relies on the practitioner not only being willing to see practice anew but to deliberately look at practice from a different viewpoint.

Critical appreciation also requires practitioners to develop their self-critical skills, to enable them to gain self-knowledge regarding their performance. These skills are difficult to acquire and self-comment often tends to be justificatory rather than critical.

Cooperative learning

Cooperative learning is very effective in promoting learning to work in teams (Biggs, 1999; Griffiths, 1999). This makes cooperative learning an essential framework for inclusion within an interprofessional learning environment.

Healthy cooperative learning has five important and necessary features (Johnson *et al.* 1998).

1. **Positive interdependence**

   Positive interdependence means being interconnected. Learners strive together to reach a common goal, with each learner's efforts being required and indispensable to the group's success. The learners 'sink or swim together' and there can be no 'free riders'. Each group member has a unique contribution to make to the joint effort because of their resources and/or role and task responsibilities. Group members provide mutual support and encouragement and celebrate their joint success together.

   An example of a common goal would be the completion of a task such as a patient problem that required a range of health and social professionals to work together to make a joint decision.

2. **Face-to-face promotive interaction**

   Promotive interaction can be defined as individuals encouraging and facilitating each other's efforts to achieve, complete tasks and produce in order to reach the group's goals. This is usually synchronous, purposeful activity such as discussion, debate and joint decision making.

3. Individual accountability

Individual accountability means that each individual is assessed for mastery of the content of a task and is held responsible for contributing a fair share to the success of the group. This is an important factor because it means that no one can opt out of learning or be allowed to hide behind the work of others.

4. Interpersonal and small-group skills

This involves teaching members of the team skills needed to succeed. In order for learners to coordinate efforts to achieve mutual goals, learners must get to know and trust each other, communicate accurately and unambiguously, accept and support each other, and resolve conflict constructively.

5. Group processing

Group processing is reflecting on the actions, both group and individual, to describe what actions were helpful and unhelpful and to make decisions about what actions to continue or change. The purpose of group processing is to clarify and improve the effectiveness of the members contributing to the collaboration efforts in order to achieve the group goals.

These five essential elements of cooperative learning promote both interprofessional teamwork and interprofessional learning within the practice environment.

Reflective activity

Think of a learning activity that is focused on providing optimal care for the patient within an interprofessional environment. Using the five essential elements of the cooperative learning model consider the following:

1. What is the common goal for the learning activity?
2. Who are the members of the interprofessional team involved in achieving the common goal?
3. What methods will be used to encourage face-to-face promotive interaction?
4. How will the individual group members and the team be assessed for their mastery of skills and contribution to the team activity?
5. How will you facilitate the development of team skills?
6. What methods will you use in the team activity to facilitate reflection on the effectiveness of the team in achieving its goals?

○━┳ *Keywords*
....

Personal knowledge

Knowledge that is acquired through experiences, either directly or vicariously, much of which does not have much apparent connection with learning.

   Personal knowledge and social knowledge are complementary, with an individual's development being the product of the transaction between personal experience and the system of social knowledge interacted with

Social knowledge

Knowledge that is created through an interaction with social, political, economical and cultural context in which the experience occurs

Collaboration

Collaboration between old-timers and newcomers within a community of practice is a key concept of situated learning. Vygotsky (1978), a Russian psychologist, identified a 'zone of proximal development' in which a learner's development occurs through participation in activities slightly beyond their competence with the assistance of more skilled practitioners. Learning takes place in the zone of proximal development via interactions between an individual's **personal knowledge** system and the **social knowledge** system.

Members of a community of practice therefore become collaborators in learning, with individuals being pushed to move beyond their current capabilities in order for new learning to occur.

Coaching

Coaching, another key aspect of an interprofessional situated-learning environment, is centred on unlocking a practitioner's potential to maximise their own performance. It models many aspects of interprofessional working, enabling health- and social-care professionals to learn about each other as they learn together.

Coaching is an ideal framework for learning as it has the adaptability to support different practitioners with different learning styles within the community of practice. A coaching relationship is one of collaboration, with the emphasis being on enabling the practitioner to fully develop their skills and to facilitate a shift in their knowledge and behaviour. Key elements of coaching include: identification of specific goals; focused learning opportunities and challenges; provision of feedback; time for reflection, analysis and action planning; and support.

McLellan describes coaching as:

> observing students [learners/practitioners] while they carry out a task, providing a 'guide on the side' who intervenes and provides scaffolding for learning to progress when necessary, but otherwise fades into the background providing learners with opportunities for initiative and self-directed problem solving: constructive learning.
>
> McLellan (1996, p. 11)

Within a community of practice, coaching provides a flexible development approach for individual practitioners that can be delivered at the right time and in parallel with the community's need to constantly change and adapt to an ever-changing environment.

Tools for learning

Reflection

Reflective practice is associated with learning from experience and as such is a key learning and teaching strategy within a situated-learning environment. Using the process of reflection within a community of practice will help to generate practice-based knowledge and offers a practice-based learning activity that not only contributes to the continuing professional development (CPD) of the individual practitioner but also to the continuing development of the community.

Reflection within the health- and social-care setting is a prerequisite to professional caring. It is an intentional activity that enables the practitioner to become more self-aware of the contradictions that exist between how we would like to practise and how we actually do. Engaging in reflective practice is associated with improving and changing practice and stimulating personal and professional growth.

Reflection has been defined by Boyd and Fales as:

> the process of internally examining and exploring an issue of concern triggered by an experience, which creates and clarifies meaning in terms of self and which results in a changed conceptual perspective.
>
> Boyd and Fales (1983, p. 100)

When we, as health- and social-care practitioners think of reflection, how do we perceive it? In one sense, reflection relates to the carrying out of a number of practices and our understanding of them, in another it relates to thoughts, feelings and understanding of particular events. But how well do we reflect, how well do we use reflection and how does the reflective process sit within a situated-learning environment?

The work of Donald Schon is widely regarded as the most seminal on the subject of reflection in professional practice. Schon (1983) identifies two types of reflection: reflection-in-action and reflection-on-action. Reflection-in-action is the process whereby the practitioner recognises a new situation or a problem and thinks about it while still acting. Reflection-on-action, on the other hand, is the retrospective contemplation of practice undertaken in order to uncover knowledge used in a particular situation, by analysing and interpreting the information recalled.

There have been a number of structured models of reflection developed to encourage practitioners to reflect on their practice, including Gibbs (1988); Atkins and Murphy (1993); Johns (1994) and Driscoll (2000).

👍 *Over to you*

Look up the models of reflection mentioned in the last paragraph and consider which one(s) you feel would provide the most appropriate strategy to guide your reflection.

The use of structured reflection models fosters a mechanistic approach towards reflection. This may result in reflection becoming cold, detached and devoid of the nature of caring, representative of technical processes as opposed to dynamic relationships, and lacking in the real representation of skilled health- and social-care practice.

If practitioners viewed their work as art, reflections on both their *practices* and *thoughts* on practice could be represented through the symbolism of art. Practitioners could look deep into their portrait of practice, considering, for example, its composition, tone, subject matter, space and form. These concepts are taken from the arts and used when critically analysing paintings (Acton, 1997). Using these concepts to reflect on practice can lead practitioners through uncovering layers of knowledge and practice, revealing the meaning of the practices, or enabling practitioners to apply layers to the existing professional practice. Practitioners' portraits of practice can be represented, for example, as stories, paintings, mime and poetry.

This approach to reflection would enable learners to develop an appreciation of the complexities of their practice and that of their community of practice.

Narratives

Narratives, when used as part of a learning and teaching strategy, can be of considerable value in both the personal and professional development of health- and social-care practitioners. So what is a narrative? Hardy writes that narrative is:

> a primary state of mind. [There is an] inner and outer story-telling that plays a major role in our sleeping and waking lives . . . for we dream in narrative, daydream in narrative, remember, anticipate, hope, despair, believe, doubt, plan, revise, criticise, gossip, learn, hate and love by narrative. In order really to live we make up stories about ourselves and other personnel as well as the social past and future.
>
> Hardy (1978, p. 12)

Health- and social-care practitioners know patients through the stories patients tell and health- and social-care practitioners respond with stories of their own. The knowledge the practitioner gains about a patient is extended into further narratives when conveyed to others. Stories are told about stories and narratives thus become a form of social interaction.

Narrative provides meaning, context and perspective for health- and social-care practice. It is a way of knowing – a discovery – which defines how, why and in what way practice is occurring. Narrative offers practitioners a possibility of understanding that cannot be arrived at by any other means. Narratives are a way in which the individual can gain personal knowledge and social knowledge, offering a learning opportunity which gives the individual the freedom to be who they are, rather than comply with the practitioner's vision of optimal practice. Biases, assumptions and prejudices are encountered so that new possibilities for connection are discovered. The use of narrative as a learning strategy to promote the humanistic dimensions of care has been used in medicine (Greenhalgh and Hurwitz, 1998), nursing (Benner *et al.*, 1996) and physiotherapy (Jenson *et al.*, 1999). Narratives are undoubtedly a learning strategy that could be used by all health- and social-care professions. As Greenhalgh and Hurwitz succinctly state:

> In the education of patients and professionals, narratives:
> - are often memorable
> - are ground in experience
> - enforce reflection.
>
> Greenhalgh and Hurwitz (1998, p. 7)

What is a narrative?
- It has a beginning, middle and end.
- It has a narrator and a listener and is thereby created in a relationship.
- The narrative is concerned with the individual.
- The choice of what to tell and what to omit lies entirely with the narrator.
- It engages the listener and invites an interpretation.
- It is a means of developing professional knowledge.

Stories have the potential to reveal what is significant and relevant to the practitioners about situations and events in their practice. Providing the practitioner with the occasion to tell their story and also to hear their story affords the practitioner the opportunity to reflect upon the paths and options that they did not take at the time and perhaps consider ones that did not occur when the event took place.

Reflective activity

Select a practice skill that a learner you are working with needs to acquire.
   Use the situated learning model to design and develop a learning environment that is suitable for the learner to acquire the practice skill. Consider the following:

- Think about which members of the community of practice will be involved in facilitating the development of the practice skill.
- Consider where in the community of practice the learning should take place.
- What learning and teaching strategies will you use and why?
- Think about the role that you will adopt within the situated activity.

Key points Top tips

The key points of a situated-learning environment are:
- that it fosters the development of lifelong learning skills
- that situated learning and teaching strategies include critical appreciation; cooperative learning; collaboration; reflection; coaching and narrative
- that learning takes place in the zone of proximal development through interactions between a newcomer and an old-timer
- that the learner and the facilitator are actively involved in and jointly manage the responsibility for learning
- situated learning techniques take more time and effort for both the learner and facilitator

How do we support learners in the practice environment?

It is essential that learners are supported within the practice environment to enable them to develop both personally and professionally. In the health- and social-care professions, this support is usually provided by a professional who takes on the role of a mentor. A mentor may also be described as a supervisor, facilitator, clinical supervisor, practice teacher, clinical lecturer or placement educator. In this section, the term 'mentor' (and the related 'mentorship') encompasses all these terms.

The literature indicates that there is a growing interest amongst all the health- and social-care professions in developing the mentorship role. The Department of Health document *Meeting the Challenge: A Strategy for the Allied Health Professionals* (Department of Health, 2000b, p. 5) states: 'supervising students is a key part of every professional practitioner's role'. The English National Board for Nursing, Midwifery and Health Visiting (ENB) and the Department of Health document *Preparation of Mentors and Teachers* (2001) discusses the importance of nursing and midwifery students receiving high-quality mentorship from practitioners. The Nursing and Midwifery Council's Code of Professional Conduct states that:

> Nurses and midwives on the NMC professional register have a duty to facilitate students of nursing and midwifery and others to develop their competence.
>
> The Nursing and Midwifery Council's Code of Professional Conduct (2004a, section 6.4)

The British Medical Association (2004) emphasises that mentoring should be available to all medical students for confidential, professional and personal advice.

Although these documents are written by specific professional bodies, the issues raised regarding the quality of mentorship and the role of the mentor are pertinent to all health- and social-care professions.

Over to you

Read your professional code of conduct. Find out what your responsibility is for facilitating students of your own profession and others to develop their competence.

History of mentoring

The term 'mentoring' originates in Greek mythology. The Greek poet Homer in his epic poem the *Odyssey* first used the word 'mentor'. In his poem, Homer tells the story of Odysseus who went away to fight the Trojan War leaving the care of his son Telemachus to his wise and trusted friend Mentor. The relationship between Mentor and Telemachus was described as nurturing, educative and protective. It ensured Telemachus's personal and social development and also that he was prepared professionally for his responsibilities and tasks ahead.

In more recent times, the idea of mentoring has attracted attention from trainers, educators, policy makers and the business world, all of them interested in initial and continuing professional development. Mentoring first became popular during the 1970s and 1980s as a method of professional development in the USA. In the late 1980s, the private sector in the UK began to take a keen interest in the potential of mentoring and in the 1990s mentoring began to cross the public–private divide.

Today, mentoring has been embraced by many diverse organisations and professions and has been described as 'a developmental alliance', occupying an important position in the initial and continuing development of many health- and social-care professionals.

What is mentoring?

Mentoring has been variously defined within and outside of the health- and social-care professions, which has led to there being no agreement on the meaning of the term. Oxley, for example, defines mentoring as:

> The process whereby an experienced, highly regarded, empathic person (the mentor), guides another individual (the mentee) in the development and re-examination of their own ideas,

learning, and personal and professional development. The mentor, who often, but not necessarily, works in the same organisation or field as the mentee, achieves this by listening and talking in confidence to the mentee.

Oxley (1998, cited in BMA, 2004, p. 3)

Other definitions include Ehrich *et al.*, (2002) who define mentoring as a 'personal helping relationship between a mentor and mentee/protégé that includes professional development and growth and varying degrees of support'. Clutterbuck (2004) defines mentoring as principally listening with empathy, mutually sharing experiences, professional friendship, developing insight through reflection and being a sounding board.

These examples highlight that the term 'mentoring' means different things to different people and as a consequence there is no agreed definition.

Mentoring as a concept, and its practice, has been widely accepted by the health- and social-care professions as being important, but the profile of a mentor varies depending on the profession. In nursing and midwifery, for example, mentoring has a high profile, with a requirement for all nursing and midwifery students to be assigned a mentor for the duration of their practice placement. To undertake the role of a mentor, nursing and midwifery practitioners must have undertaken a mentorship programme or equivalent, which is approved by the Nursing and Midwifery Council (NMC). In addition, to remain a mentor, mentors are required to attend and record an annual mentor update. In contrast, within social work the mentor has a low profile. This may be because many of the characteristics and functions of mentoring have traditionally been included within the role of the social-work supervisor.

What is the role of a mentor?

Within the literature a mentor is defined by the various roles that the mentor, undertakes. I would like to suggest the following definition for a mentor which encompasses all the roles: an experienced professional who teaches, supports, advises, guides, acts as a resource and role model and promotes self-development, fulfilment of potential and confidence in the learner (mentee) achieving both professional and life goals.

Within health- and social-care professions, definitions of a mentor tend to emphasise facilitation of learning above other mentoring roles and include the role of an assessor. For example, the Nursing and Midwifery Council (NMC) define a mentor as:

> A mentor is a nurse, midwife or specialist community public health nurse who facilitates learning and supervises and assesses students in a practice setting.

NMC (2005)

There is no single personality type that is synonymous with that of being or becoming an effective mentor. You can find, within the literature, an extensive range of characteristics or qualities which students consider to be essential in a good mentor. These have been listed in Table 6.1 under headings regarding the roles undertaken by a mentor. This list is by no means exhaustive and is not presented in any particular order.

Table 6.1 Qualities students consider important in a mentor

Personal qualities	• Enthusiastic, friendly, approachable • Patient and understanding • Sense of humour • Non-judgemental, tolerant and accepts personal differences.
Role model	• Organised • Able to set a good example • Confident and secure with self, cares about others and treats everyone with respect.
Teacher	• Effective communicator • Knowledgeable and up to date in their field • Able to help with goal setting and planning • Willing to share personal experiences, knowledge and skills • Good source of information.
Guide/supervisor	• Able to encourage personal and professional development • Able to instil confidence and motivate people • Proactive, imaginative and creative • Open to other points of view • Realistic expectations of the student • Able to know when to give and when not to give advice • Able to act as a friend while at the same time providing guidance.
Assessor	• Prepared to use constructive criticism • Provides regular feedback on the student's performance.

Mentors have a pivotal role to play in the delivery of the next generation of health- and social-care professionals. Those mentors involved in supporting pre-registration students have a responsibility to ensure that the student is fit for purpose, fit for practice and fit for award before the student gains their licence to practice from the appropriate regulatory body, for example the Nursing and Midwifery Council, or Health Professions Council. Mentors therefore act as gatekeepers to their profession and take responsibility for protecting the public.

Health professional speaks

Naveen, an experienced community nurse and mentor, speaks of her experiences as a mentor.

Although initially I felt that I had little choice in becoming a mentor, on reflection it has been a thoroughly worthwhile experience, although frustrating at times. The challenge has always been attempting to juggle patient needs, team management, course requirements and student expectations all at the same time! However, over the nine years of being a mentor within the community setting the rewards have much outweighed those difficulties.

The greatest satisfaction comes from students coming back to your area year on year as this enables you to see how they are progressing, not only in skills and competence, but also in self-belief that they can actually achieve their goal of becoming a registered nurse. Seeing staff nurses in the corridor in the local hospital who still remember you as their mentor, hopefully fondly, or students who had not thought of a community nursing career return to community nursing posts once qualified is fantastic. It's nice to think that maybe I, in some small way, might have made a difference to that student.

Evidence base

Read *Guidance for Mentors of Student Nurses and Midwives: An RCN toolkit* (Royal College of Nursing, 2005).
Although this toolkit has been designed for mentors of student nurses and midwives, much of the information included is relevant to mentors of students from all health- and social-care professions.

Reflective activity

Think about a health- or social-care practitioner who has been your mentor. Consider the following:

- What do you feel were the strengths and weaknesses of your mentor?
- How did your mentor's strengths and weaknesses influence the quality of your learning experience while you were assigned to your mentor?
- As a learner, how could you have improved this mentor–learner relationship?

Interprofessional mentorship

As we have seen, mentorship has a long history, but the concept of interprofessional mentorship is relatively new and in its infancy in health- and social-care professions. It is essential that learners are supported appropriately within interprofessional situated-learning environments. Interprofessional mentorship would appear to be the way ahead for supporting learners.

What is interprofessional mentorship?

At the current time, the literature relating to mentors and mentorship reveals only one definition of interprofessional mentorship. Marshall and Gordon define interprofessional mentorship as:

> Occasions when a health or social care professional facilitates interprofessional learning and supervises and assesses students in the practice setting.
>
> Marshall and Gordon (2005, p. 39)

The focus of interprofessional mentorship, therefore, is to facilitate learning opportunities for students to enable them to learn from and with professionals from their own and other professions in the practice setting. The patient is always at the centre of the interprofessional learning experience, with the overall aim being to improve collaboration between different professional groups and the quality of care. Thus, interprofessional mentorship will focus on the facilitation of the knowledge, skills and understanding required to work successfully within the interprofessional context.

What are the key characteristics of an interprofessional mentor?

Earlier in this chapter we identified the key characteristics of a mentor, which included effective communication and interpersonal skills, being enthusiastic, friendly, approachable, organised, patient, understanding, caring, knowledgeable and up to date in their field, able to help with goal setting and planning, and acting as a good source of information (see Table 6.1 on page 125).

If we review these key characteristics of a uniprofessional mentor, it can be seen that these are generic rather than profession-specific skills. It would therefore be possible for mentors to transfer these skills to situations involving learners from different professional groups. This would make interprofessional mentorship a possibility for all mentors and all learners, regardless of the professional background.

What is the role of an interprofessional mentor?

The primary roles of an interprofessional mentor are the same as those of a uniprofessional mentor, that is, the facilitation of learning, supervision and assessment of learners in the practice environment. The application of these roles, however, would be related to the learner's interprofessional learning outcomes.

Learners currently have profession-specific interprofessional learning outcomes articulated, as well as profession-specific learning outcomes.

These learning outcomes can be found in the relevant professional, regulatory and statutory bodies' documentation. For example, Quality Assurance Agency benchmark statements (QAA, 2001); *Standards of Proficiency for Pre-registration Nursing Education* (NMC, 2004b); *Standards of Proficiency for Pre-registration Midwifery Education* (NMC, 2004c); Good Medical Practice (GMC, 2001); *Standards of Proficiency: Radiographers* (HPC, 2003).

It would, however, be beneficial to have interprofessional learning outcomes that were applicable to all health- and social-care learners. This would provide a common framework for the development of interprofessional learning, teaching and assessment. The Combined Universities Interprofessional Learning Unit has developed an interprofessional capability framework (CUILU, 2004). The overall aim of this framework is to describe the capabilities that any undergraduate student of health- and social care is required to achieve in order to become a capable interprofessional worker. The framework has been divided into four key areas: knowledge in practice, ethical practice, interprofessional working, and reflection (learning).

At the time of writing, the interprofessional capability framework was a working document to be further developed and validated by a process of collaborative inquiry by students and practitioners. This framework provides those involved in delivering interprofessional learning with a tool for identifying new approaches in collaborative learning and working within a range of practice contexts. In addition, the framework can provide a focus for the assessment of learning outcomes that might be met by a learner spending time with a practitioner from another profession.

Evidence base

Look at the website www.cuilu.group./shef.ac.uk/ and locate the interprofessional capability framework.

RRRRRapid recap

Check your progress so far by working through each of the following questions.

1. What are the key features of a community of practice?
2. List the key points of situated learning theory.
3. What are the key features of a situated-learning environment?
4. What is the role of an interprofessional mentor?

If you have difficulty with more than one of the questions, read through the section again to refresh your understanding before moving on.

References

Acton, M. (1997) *Learning to Look at Paintings.* Routledge, London.

Atkins, S. and Murphy, K. (1993) Reflection: A Review of the Literature. *Journal of Advanced Nursing,* **10**(0): 1100–1192.

Benner, P., Tanner, C.A. and Chesla, C.A. (1996) *Expertise in Nursing Practice.* Springer, New York.

Biggs, J. (1999) *Teaching for Quality Learning at University: What the Student Does?* Society for Research into Higher Education and Open University Press, Buckingham.

British Medical Association (2004) *Exploring Mentoring.* BMA, London. Available from: www.bma.org.uk/ap.nsf/Content/Mentoring/$file/mentoring.pdf.

Boyd, E.M. and Fales, A.W. (1983) Reflective Learning: Key to Learning from Experience. *Journal of Humanistic Psychology,* **23**: 99–117.

Clutterbuck, D. (2004) *Everybody Needs a Mentor.* Chartered Institute of Personnel Development, London.

CUILU (2004) *The Interprofessional Capability Framework.* Available from: www.cuilu.group./shef.ac.uk/

Department of Health (1999) *Making a Difference: Strengthening the Nursing, Midwifery and Health Visiting Contribution to Health and Health care.* Department of Health, London. Available from: www.dh.gov.uk/publications.

Department of Health (2000a) *The NHS Plan: A Plan for Investment, a Plan for Reform.* Department of Health, London. Available from: www.dh.gov.uk/publications.

Department of Health (2000b) *Meeting the Challenge: A Strategy for the Allied Health Professions.* Department of Health, London. Available from: www.dh.gov.uk/publications.

Department of Health (2000c) *A Health Service of all the Talents: Developing the NHS Workforce.* Department of Health, London. Available from: www.dh.gov.uk/publications.

Department of Health (2001) *Working Together, Learning Together: A Framework for Lifelong Learning for the NHS.* Department of Health, London. Available from: www.dh.gov.uk/PublicationsAndStatistics/Publications/PublicationsPolicyAndGuidance/PublicationsPolicyAndGuidanceArticle/fs/en?CONTENT_ID=4009558&chk=tCWmaW.

Department of Health (2002) Next Steps in Joint Training for Health Professionals. Press Release: Reference number 2002/0078. Available from: www.dh.gov.uk/PublicationsAndStatistics/PressReleases/fs/en.

Department of Health and Social Security (1974) *Report of the Committee of Enquiry into the Care and Supervision Provided in Relation to Maria Colwell.* HMSO, London.

Department for Education and Skills (2005) *Common Core Skills and Knowledge for the Children's Workforce.* DfES Publications, London. Available from http://publications.teachernet.gov.uk/.

Driscoll, J. (2000) *Practising Clinical Supervision: A Reflective Approach.* Bailliere Tindall, London.

Ehrich, L., Tennet, L. and Hansford, B. (2002) A review of mentoring in education: Some Lessons for Nursing. *Contemporary Nurse,* **12**(3); 253–264.

English National Board for Nursing, Midwifery and Health Visiting and Department of Health (2001) *Preparation of Mentors and Teachers.* ENB and Department of Health, London.

Fish, D. (1989) *Appreciating Practice in the Caring Professions: Re-focusing Professional Development and Practitioner Research.* Butterworth-Heinemann, Oxford.

General Medical Council (2001) Good Medical Practice. GMC, London.

Gibbs, G. (1998) *Learning by Doing: A Guide to Teaching and Learning Methods.* Further Education Unit, Oxford Brookes University, Oxford.

Greenhalgh, T. and Hurwitz, B. (1998) *Narrative Based Medicine: Dialogue and Discourse in Clinical Practice.* BMJ Books, London.

Griffiths, S. (1999) Teaching and Learning in Small Groups. In *A Handbook for Teaching and Learning in Higher Education: Enhancing Academic Practice* (eds. Fry, H., Ketteridge, S. and Marshall, S.). Kogan Page, London, pp. 95–107.

Hardy, B. (1978) Narrative as a Primary Act of Mind. In *The Cool Web: The Patterns of Children's Reading* (eds. Meek, M., Warlow, A. and Barton, G.). Atheneum, New York, pp. 12–23.

Health Professional Council (2003) *Standards of Proficiency: Radiographers.* HPC, London.

Jenson, G.M., Shephard, K.F., Gywer, J. and Hack, L.M. (1999) *Expertise in Physical Therapy Practice.* Butterworth Heinemann, USA.

Johns, C. (1994) Guided Reflection. In *Reflective Practice in Nursing* (ed. Palmer, A.). Blackwell Science, Oxford.

Johnson, D., Johnson W., Roger T. and Smith K.A. (1998) *Active Learning Cooperation in the Classroom.* Interaction Book Company, Edina.

Lave, J. (1988) *Cognition in Practice.* Cambridge University Press, Cambridge.

Lave, J. and Wenger, E. (1991) *Situated Learning – Legitimate Peripheral Participation.* Cambridge University Press, Cambridge.

Marshall, M. and Gordon, F. (2005) Interprofessional Mentorship: Taking on the Challenge. *Journal of Integrated Care,* **13**(2): 38–41.

McLellan, H. (1996) *Situated Learning Perspectives.* Educational Technology Publications, Englewood Cliffs.

Nursing and Midwifery Council (2004a) *Code of Professional Conduct: Standards for Conduct, Performance and Ethics.* NMC, London.

Nursing and Midwifery Council (2004b*) Standards of Proficiency for Pre-Registration Nursing Education.* NMC, London.

Nursing and Midwifery Council (2004c) *Standards of Proficiency for Pre-Registration Midwifery Education.* NMC, London.

Nursing and Midwifery Council (2005) *NMC Consultation on a Standard to Support Learning and Assessment in Practice, Final Report.* NMC, London.

Quality Assurance Agency for Higher Education (2001) *Benchmark Statements: Health care Programmes.* QAA, Gloucester. Available from: www.qaa.ac.uk/academicinfrastructure/benchmark/health.

Rogoff, B. (1990) *Apprenticeship in Thinking: Cognitive Development in Social Context.* Oxford University Press, Oxford.

Royal College of Nursing (2005) *Guidance for Mentors of Student Nurses and Midwives: An RCN Toolkit.* RCN, London.

Schon, D. (1983) *The Reflective Practitioner: How Professionals Think in Action.* Basic Books, New York.

Secretary of State for Health (2001) *Learning from Bristol.* The Stationery Office, London.

Secretary of State for Health (2003) *The Victoria Climbié Inquiry.* The Stationery Office, London.

University of Salford (2004) Education and Training for Interagency Working: New Standards. Available from www.chssc.salford.ac.uk/scswr.

Vygotsky, L.S. (1978) *Mind in Society. The Development of Higher Psychological Processes.* Harvard University Press, Cambridge, MA.

Zwarenstein M., Reeves S., Barr H., Hammick M., Koppel I. and Atkins J. (2001) Interprofessional education: effects on professional practice and health care outcomes (Cochrane Review). Available from The Cochrane Library, Oxford.

7

Barriers to effective interprofessional working

Learning outcomes

By the end of this chapter you should be able to:

★ Identify the barriers to effective interprofessional working

★ Critically assess the impact that the identified barriers have on providing effective health- and social-care delivery

★ Be aware of the differing professional, regulatory and statutory requirements which impact on the interprofessional approach to the exercise of duty of care.

The barriers to successful interprofessional working

In previous chapters, we have considered the essential factors which, if considered as a whole, contribute towards effective interprofessional working.

These factors include:

● UK health- and social-care policies and legislation
● Teams, teamwork and team dynamics
● Leadership and expertise
● Communicating with each other
● Interprofessional learning.

It is now recognised that a single profession or individual can no longer deliver the complex patient care that is demanded in the 21st century. Interprofessional collaboration is essential to the successful achievement of an integrated care system that will enhance patient outcome. Changes in the structure and functioning of the NHS are taking place to facilitate interprofessional collaboration. For example, single interprofessional patient records, and multidisciplinary team meetings (MDT meetings).

Periods of change are, however, uncomfortable and frequently meet with resistance. The transition towards interprofessional working is no exception and it is important to identify the problems, issues and needs that may arise during this period of change. D'Amour and Oandasan (2005) identified three elements that determine how collaboration develops and is consolidated in health care teams:

1. **Systemic factors** – conditions outside the organisation
2. **Organisational factors** – conditions within the organisation
3. **Interactional factors** – interpersonal relationships between team members.

The environment in which interprofessional collaboration takes place is influenced by systemic factors. In a professional practice setting, two of the elements are operating: the organisation (organisational factors) and the team (interactional factors). The dynamics of interprofessional collaboration are influenced by all three elements (Martin-Rodriguez *et al.* 2005).

In this final chapter, we will use these three elements to explore the potential barriers that exist to successful interprofessional collaboration and explore practical solutions to removing these barriers.

Systemic factors

Systemic factors are those factors outside of the organisation that impact, either negatively or positively, on interprofessional working. These factors include the professional system and the social system.

The professional system

The professional system has a significant impact on the development of effective interprofessional working. This is because the professional system appears to run counter to the philosophy of collaboration. In this section, we will consider a number of different aspects of the professional system including:

- professional socialisation
- professional language
- professional tribes and territories
- professional codes of conduct
- professions and professionalisation.

Professional socialisation

Professional socialisation has been defined by Merton *et al.* as:

> the process by which people selectively acquire the values and attitudes, the interests, skills and knowledge – in short, the culture – current in groups of which they are, or seek to become a member.
>
> Merton *et al.* (1959, cited in Clouder, 2003 p. 213)

Early studies of professional socialisation describe a process whereby health- and social-care students are shaped and moulded into 'good' or 'ideal' professionals. This suggests that the student is a passive recipient of knowledge and skills and internalises the profession's culture completely, without question.

Today, however, a different approach is taken to professional socialisation, which is based on 'socialisation as interaction' (Clouder, 2003). This view on professional socialisation suggests that a student enters the social world of a profession and, through face-to-face communication with others, establishes what it is to be a professional. The profession has a structure that is created by the way in which members of the profession structure its activities. This structure may, however, be modified over time as new shared understandings are negotiated through the process of professional socialisation of newcomers, for example students. In this approach to professional socialisation the student is not passive but is actively using their personal experience to shape their perceptions of their profession.

The process of professional socialisation begins as soon as a student enters their professional education programme. The student becomes immersed in the philosophies, values and theoretical perspectives inherent in their profession. Each profession is established on different philosophies, values and theoretical bases. Within an interprofessional team, these differences between the various professionals are potential sources of conflict and as a consequence may hinder the development of effective interprofessional working. Table 7.1 illustrates the values, philosophies and theoretical differences of members of an interprofessional team.

Table 7.1 The values, philosophies and theoretical differences of members of an interprofessional team

	Doctors	Nurses	Social workers
Values	● Advocate saving life	● Advocate humanism	● Advocate quality of life
Questions asked by professionals	● Disease oriented. E.g. What is the diagnosis? What is the prognosis? What are the symptoms?	● Patient oriented. E.g. What will help this patient to function as well as possible? What support does this patient have at home?	● Groups or individual clients e.g. What services are available for elderly clients? What social services does this client need?
Treatments and management goals for the patient/client	● Based on the medical model. Identifying signs and symptoms. Diagnosing the disease. Treating the disease. Curing the disease.	● Based on the health/ illness model. Identifying the patient's health/illness needs. Helping the patient with the activities of daily living. Interested in the holistic view of the patient.	● Based on psycho-social model. Using personality and social resources to improve the situation.
Professional expectations	● Expert ● Full responsibility for care of patient ● Leader.	● Supportive, nurturing ● Teaching, mentoring ● Enabling of self-direction ● Makes a difference ● Teamwork.	● Trustworthy ● Shared responsibility ● Active listener ● Honest ● Reliable.

Solutions

A strategy that could be used to overcome this potential source of conflict is for each profession to be explicit about its philosophy and to be prepared to share its values beyond the confines of its professional boundaries. Time should be set aside at team meetings for team members to explore and discuss their different philosophies, values and theoretical bases. Open discussion of differing perspectives can act as a stimulus for new questions and development of the team. This will help the team members to recognise and value the diversity that the different professionals bring to the team. The team will then be able to build on each other's strengths and work together more effectively.

Differences in professional language

Different professional groups use language very differently. Even when different professions use the same words, the words may mean different things. For example, the term 'service user' may refer to a patient, a client, the family, other service agencies or the community in general. Another example is the term 'assessment'. Assessments are carried out by community nurses, doctors and social workers but the process, context and outcome is very different to each of the professions.

Differences in professional language create a real challenge to the development of collaboration and successful interprofessional working. It means that communication is hindered as the professionals may not be able to understand each other or alternatively they may believe they have understood each other, when actually their interpretations of the conversations are very different as a result of the different meanings that have been attached to specific words.

Unless different professionals are able to effectively communicate with each other, interprofessional working and hence integrated care will not become a reality.

Solutions

- **Interprofessional education**. Interprofessional education provides an opportunity for all health- and social-care professionals to discover that different professions may use language very differently. Learners will be able to develop an understanding of the language from the perspective of the different professionals. At the same time, the learner will be able to clarify the meaning of words from their own profession.

- **Develop a common language**. Another strategy is for the team to decide on a common language/common terminology that the team are going to use. This will involve the team identifying terms that mean something different to different professional groups. The team will then need to explore and discuss the terms before agreeing on a common definition for each. A good example would be the one given above, relating to assessment. If the team wished to introduce an interprofessional assessment tool, the team would first have to come to a common definition for assessment, which was understood by all team members.

Professional tribes and territories

Interprofessional working is seen by some professionals as a threat to their professional identity, fearing that traditional boundaries between health- and social-care professionals will disappear. When we feel under attack, our natural reaction is to retreat into our professional tribe within boundaries and territory with which we are familiar. This may be a natural reaction to conflict and change – resist and defend your tribe at all costs – but it is important that health- and social-care professionals are able to make this transition and are, thus, able to effectively collaborate within an interprofessional team.

So what is a tribe? As people banded together to constitute primitive societies thousands of years ago, the first major form of organisation to emerge was the tribe. The tribe's key function was to infuse a distinct sense of social identity and belonging, thereby strengthening people's ability to bond and survive as individuals and as a collective. A classic tribe may be tied to a specific territory and the exploitation of resources found there. In different tribes, the members speak different languages, practice different rituals and may share some language and rituals with members of other tribes. If we consider this definition of a classic tribe we can see that the notion of 'tribes' and 'tribalism' are useful metaphors when discussing health- and social-care professions.

Within the definition of a classic tribe, territory is mentioned.

A territory refers to an area in which one has rights and responsibilities. Sometimes the area is a concrete space, for example a ward or department; sometimes it is a sphere of knowledge; and sometimes it refers to elements of both (Dombeck, 1997). Think about how you would introduce yourself at an interprofessional meeting, you might say, for example:

> I am Arijeta, I am a senior therapeutic radiographer working in the oncology department at this hospital.

> I am Rageh, a third-year nursing student on placement in the oncology ward at this hospital.

In these introductions, both Arijeta and Rageh have described themselves in terms of who they are, their profession, their place of work, and their position within an organisation. As Arijeta and Rageh are introducing themselves, they are also staking out their territories and their boundaries. It is therefore not surprising that territorial and tribal issues arise in interprofessional practice.

Solutions

- **Articulating professional identity**. It is important that individual professionals know and are able to articulate their own professional identity before engaging with interprofessional working. It is difficult to work collaboratively if you are unsure of your own professional identity. Individual professionals must consider what their unique contribution to the interprofessional team is, both as a professional and as a person. For example, what unique knowledge, skills, and professional and personal qualities do you as a nurse, radiographer, midwife, social worker or physiotherapist bring to the interprofessional team and thus to the care and management of patients. If professionals are able to articulate their uniqueness, they will feel less threatened when collaborating with other professionals.

- **Interprofessional working**. It is important that interprofessional working is seen as integrated working and not as a blurring or dismantling of traditional professional boundaries. Integrated working and hence interprofessional working is concerned with different professionals sharing tasks and common skills if there is overlap between the roles of different professional groups, while at the same time each individual retaining their unique combination of skills.

The success of interprofessional working depends on the team identifying clear and distinct boundaries regarding what tasks to share (based upon common skills and tasks), on what occasions, to what effect and where (Rushmer and Pallis, 2002). If the team is able to identify these boundaries then the team will be able to work successfully as an interprofessional team

Clear boundaries will create trust and respect between the professionals within the team. An appreciation of professional uniqueness and an awareness of crossover and overlap in knowledge and skills will also be developed if boundaries are clearly defined.

A team that does not establish clear boundaries around the areas of overlap will lead to ambiguity for the team. Among the team members, there is likely to be role uncertainty, role ambiguity, feelings of inequity, stress and anxiety and a feeling of being unprepared for the role they are expected to carry out. This lack of clarity will hinder successful interprofessional working (Rushmer and Pallis, 2002).

Reflective activity

Identify the unique contribution that both you and your profession bring to an interprofessional team. Use the following headings to help guide your thinking:

- Knowledge
- Skills
- Professional qualities
- Personal qualities.

Evidence base

Find out more about the theory of integrated working by reading the following paper:

Rushmer, R. and Pallis, G. (2002) 'Interprofessional Working: The Wisdom of Integrated Working and The Disaster of Blurred Boundaries'. *Public Money and Management,* October–December, p. 59–66.

 Case study

Delivery of effective care involving different health- and social-care professionals

A 75-year-old man, living alone, fell on a Saturday afternoon while leaving the local village shop. The owner of the shop dialled 999 and the man was admitted to hospital. The man was diagnosed with a hip fracture, which was fixed surgically. He was fit to be discharged after 10 days.

With reference to the case study:

- List the health- and social-care professionals that are most suited to providing each aspect of care for this patient.

- For each health- and social-care professional listed, identify the unique contribution that they make to the care needs of this patient.

- Identify the overlaps in the roles and responsibilities of the health- and social-care professionals' providing care for this patient.

- Discuss how the team might allocate the common/shared tasks and responsibilities between the professionals within the team.

Professional codes of conduct

Professional codes of conduct, often referred to as professional codes of ethics, are frequently cited as potential barriers to interprofessional working. But is this just a myth or is it a reality?

A code of conduct provides explicit guidance to the professional on what sorts of conduct are considered to be ethically appropriate within the sphere of professional practice (Hewison and Sim, 1998).

The existence of a code of conduct is often regarded as a prerequisite to acceptance as a profession. This makes the code of conduct an integral part of the professional system. It has been suggested that codes of conduct serve the interests of the profession itself as well as protecting the interests of those whom the profession serves. If this is the case, the codes are promoting professional exclusivity and professional distinctiveness, which may potentially compromise interprofessional working. If we review various codes of conduct we can see that they do contain statements of professional self-interest, for example:

> You must always make sure that your behaviour does not damage your profession's reputation.
>
> Health Professions Council (HPC) (2003, Standard 16)

You must uphold and enhance the good reputation of the professions.

Nursing and Midwifery Council (NMC) (2002, Section 1.2)

Social care workers must uphold public trust and confidence in social care services.

General Social Care Council (GSCC) (2002, Section 5)

You must not behave in a way, in work or outside work, which would call into question your suitability to work in social care services.

GSCC (2002, Section 5.1)

However, despite these statements, which clearly demonstrate professional self-interest, the codes do explicitly address cooperation and collaboration between the different health- and social-care professions, for example:

Working openly and co-operatively with colleagues and treating them with respect.

GSCC (2002, Section 6.5)

Recognising and respecting the roles and expertise of workers from other agencies and working in partnership with them.

GSCC (2002, Section 6.7)

You are expected to work co-operatively within teams and to respect the skills, expertise and contributions of your colleagues. You must treat them fairly and without discrimination.

NMC (2002, Section 4.2)

You must communicate effectively and share your knowledge, skill and expertise with other members of the team as required for the benefit of patients and clients.

NMC (2002, Section 4.3)

You must also communicate effectively, co-operate and share your knowledge and expertise with professional colleagues for the benefit of patients, clients and users.

HPC (2003, Standard 7)

When working in a team you must:
- Respect the skills and contributions of your colleagues.
- Communicate effectively with colleagues within and outside the team.

GMC (2001, Standard 36)

Professional codes of conduct do, therefore, seem to be providing a firm foundation for effective interprofessional working. In fact, if the codes are viewed in their totality, they reveal very similar aims, values and guidelines. This suggests that the areas of convergence of opinion far outweigh views that would provide a focus for conflict (Hewison and Sim, 1998). So, perhaps it is just a myth that the codes are compromising interprofessional working.

Professions and professionalisation

By definition, belonging to a profession and the process of **professionalisation** potentially inhibit the development of collaborative practice.

So how is a profession defined? Professions tend to have certain qualities in common:

- Membership of the profession is usually restricted and regulated by a professional association, for example Nursing and Midwifery Council (NMC), Health Professions Council (HPC), General Social Care Council (GSCC).
- Professions usually have a great deal of autonomy, setting rules and enforcing discipline themselves.
- Professions are generally exclusive, for example you cannot practice nursing, radiography, medicine, social work without being registered with a professional body.
- Members of a profession receive an extensive period of education and training prior to practising.
- Professions have an explicit code of conduct for practice.
- Professions have a philosophy of public service and altruism.

If we consider these common qualities of a profession, it can be seen that the concept of a profession is promoting exclusivity, territorial boundaries and distinctiveness. These factors are diametrically opposed to the factors that promote interprofessional working.

Historically, there were only three professions: medicine, law and ministry. Nursing and social work were categorised as semi-professions because of perceived limitations of their knowledge base, training and autonomy (Etzioni, 1969).

As we move towards interprofessional working, it is this hierarchy, created by categorising the professional groups into professions (higher professions) and semi professions (lower professions), that is having a significant impact on the development of collaborative practice.

The social system

Equality between professionals is one of the basic requirements of collaborative practice. However, within the health- and social-care professions power differences exist between the different professions. These power differences are most acute between the nursing and medical professions and are based on gender stereotypes and different social status. The boundaries between the nursing and medical

Keywords

Professionalisation

Is the process by which an occupation elevates itself to the level of profession professions can be traced back to when these professions emerged. In the 19th century, the medical and nursing professions evolved separately for reasons bound up with the class divisions and gender barriers of Victorian Britain. The result was that, traditionally, medicine has been dominated by males from the higher socio-economic classes, while nursing has been dominated by females from the middle socio-economic classes.

Today, the picture is different. The gender mix of these two professions has changed, for example at each level of the medical hierarchy women now make up a higher proportion than they did 10 years ago, and this trend is likely to accelerate (Salvage and Smith, 2000). In nursing, there are now proportionally more men entering the profession. The profession of nursing has also changed substantially, with nurses now taking on new and different roles and responsibilities, for example the introduction of nurse consultants, nurse specialists and nurse prescribing.

Despite these changes, however, the nurse–doctor relationship still remains problematic. It is apparent that the power imbalance, arising from gender stereotypes, is preventing effective collaboration between doctors and nurses (Zelek and Phillips, 2003; Reeves and Lewin, 2004; Salvage and Smith, 2000).

It is crucial that nurses are considered equal partners with doctors if collaborative relationships are to be established.

Organisational factors

The organisational setting may help or hinder interprofessional collaboration. In this section, we will consider the organisational factors that are potential barriers to effective collaboration within health- and social-care settings. These factors include: organisational structure, organisational philosophy, styles of leadership, team resources, methods of communication, and schedules and professional routines.

Organisational structure

Organisational changes have a tendency to reflect changes in the environment that have been triggered by wider social, political and economic changes. As a result, organisations develop at different rates and in doing so create structures, boundaries, finances, timescales and priorities that reflect their role and function (Lupton and Khan, 1998).

Historically the NHS has been based on a traditional hierarchical structure. Successful integrated care relies on successful collaboration between health- and social-care professionals and this can only occur if the traditional hierarchical structure of the NHS is replaced with a more horizontal structure. Progress towards a more horizontal structure has occurred since 1997, since the publication of the White Paper *The New*

NHS Modern, Dependable (Secretary of State for Health, 1997) but there has been some resistance to these changes by those professions that previously held powerful positions within the hierarchical structure.

Horizontal structures facilitate shared decision-making and open and direct communication, which are important factors in developing teamwork and thus fostering effective interprofessional collaboration.

Lack of organisational philosophy

It is important that the organisation's philosophy supports interprofessional collaboration among health- and social-care professionals. For example, a philosophy that values participation, open and direct communication, fairness, diversity and **interdependence** is crucial for the development of effective collaboration within health- and social-care teams (Henneman *et al.* 1995).

Ineffective leader

Team leaders can make or break a team. When developing an interprofessional team the team leader must specifically be able to:

- convey the vision of collaborative practice to the team members
- motivate the individual team members to engage in collaborative practice
- create an environment within which collaborative practice will flourish.

For a complete list of all the factors that make a team leader effective, you should refer to Chapter 4. Also in Chapter 4 we identified that the leadership style most suitable for an interprofessional team leader was a combination of leadership styles, those being transactional and transformational.

If a team leader is ineffective, the team will eventually cease to function as a team. The team members will no longer be committed to the team's shared common goals and objectives and, as a consequence, the delivery of care to patients may become fragmented.

Solutions: The selection of an appropriate team leader

It is important that a team leader is selected for his or her leadership skills rather than on the basis of status, hierarchy or availability. If this approach is taken to the selection of the team leader, the development of collaboration within an interprofessional team should be assured.

Lack of team resource

Lack of resources for the team will make it more difficult to develop effective interprofessional working. For example, sufficient time needs to be made available to enable team members to share information, develop interprofessional relationships and address team issues. A lack of available time may lead to the team not developing as effectively as it

---

⊙━╖ *Keywords*

Interdependence

Is the occurrence of a reliance on interactions among professionals whereby each is dependant on the other to accomplish their goals and tasks might. This is because both time and energy are required by all the team members to create a climate in which teamwork will flourish.

Space also needs to be made available. It is important that the team have space in which to meet for both formal and informal occasions. For example, a meeting room with all the appropriate facilities should be available for team meetings, audit meetings and multidisciplinary team (MDT) meetings. Ideally there should also be a shared rest room/coffee room where members of the team can meet informally. If there is a lack of space, it will be difficult for members of the team to communicate face to face. Also, the opportunity for mutual support, trust and respect to develop among the team members will be considerably reduced if there are no spaces available for meeting.

Solutions

- **Regular team meetings**. Team meetings should be held on a regular basis to provide an opportunity for the team leaders and members to meet and communicate face to face about matters that affect the team. Commitment to attending a team meeting is higher if the meeting has a regular 'slot' in the calendar. If staff know that the team meeting is held on the first Tuesday of the month between 2.00 p.m. and 3.30 p.m., then team members can schedule their other work commitments around the meeting (see Chapter 5 for further details on team meetings).

- **Allocation of dedicated space**. Space is often at a premium within organisations, but it is extremely important that an organisation gives consideration to providing space-sharing opportunities to health- and social-care professionals working in the same team.

Inadequate communication mechanisms

Lack of standardised documentation, for example patient records; lack of interprofessional standards, policies and protocols; and lack of formal meetings involving all team members, for example team meetings, will inhibit the development of collaboration within interprofessional teams.

Solutions

Single patient record

The implementation of electronic, interprofessional single patient records will significantly enhance collaborative practice and patient care and treatment (see Chapter 5 for further details on electronic patient records).

Standardised pro forma

The introduction of a standard multidisciplinary team (MDT) pro forma for recording the decisions made about a patient's treatment and management at the MDT meeting means that all the appropriate information is consistently recorded.

> ## *Reflective activity*
>
> Think about the interprofessional team in which you are currently working and consider the following points:
>
> ● Identify and read your team's/organisation's interprofessional standards policies and protocols.
>
> ● Identify the documentation that your team use that is unified and standardised for all professionals to use.
>
> ● Can you identify any documentation that is not standardised? If you can, develop a standardised document that could be used by all professionals within your team.

Differences in schedules and professional routines

Different professions differ in the arrangements adopted to accomplish their work and the way in which they work, which can create a barrier to effective interprofessional working. Differences in the length of the working day may prevent members of the interprofessional team attending meetings. For example, GPs plan their time around the needs of patients, and thus hold surgeries in the morning and the afternoon into the evening. GPs, therefore, would not be able to attend meetings during surgery times. As the majority of meetings are held during 'normal' working hours, that is, 9.00 a.m. to 5.00 p.m., this would preclude GPs from attending the majority of meetings.

Different professionals also work to different timescales to complete specific tasks. GPs, for example, may work quickly and make a number of assessments and decisions for their patients each day. However, a social worker may undertake long-term casework with a small number of clients. This may also result in interprofessional misunderstanding and conflict.

Solutions

Videoconferencing

It is difficult to suggest a realistic solution to this barrier to interprofessional working. One possible solution may be to use videoconferencing for team meetings. This resource is invaluable as it allows for team members, who are not located on the same sites, to participate in the team meeting without the restrictions on time from travelling.

Interactional factors

Collaboration is a process that occurs between individuals. Therefore, ultimately, it does not matter whether the government or the organisations or the professions want interprofessional working to happen, it is only those individuals involved who can determine whether or not it will happen. Good interpersonal relationships between members of the interprofessional team are, therefore, essential if collaboration is going to occur. Interactional factors that can potentially create barriers for effective interprofessional working are as follows.

Professional stereotyping

A stereotype is a rigid set of shared beliefs we have about other people because they belong to a particular group (Woods, 2000). In stereotyping, information is limited to some highly visible aspect of a person such as age, sex, race, nationality, occupation or physical appearance. This information generates judgements about what any person belonging to that given group is like and that all people belonging to that given group possess the same characteristics (Gross *et al.* 2000).

Stereotypes provide us with a mental image of a person that does not correspond to that individual but to what we infer about that individual. Very often our stereotypes are reinforced by the media, for example by films, books, music, computer games and television. Stereotypes of health- and social-care professionals may be reinforced by television programmes, such as *Casualty*, *Holby City* or *ER*.

Although stereotyping is often viewed as something that is socially undesirable, they are a human process used by everyone and may have both negative and positive outcomes. Stereotypes can lead to very damaging, negative outcomes for both health- and social-care professionals and their patients, for example discrimination may lead to an inability to really know your patient/client, which may mean that you cannot provide quality care for them; this could lead to litigation or dissatisfaction with your chosen profession. Alternatively, stereotypes can be seen as a valid mechanism whereby individuals make sense of their interactions with other groups and may be used to positively guide intergroup behaviours (Haslam *et al.* 2000). It is this positive outcome of stereotyping that health- and social-care professionals need to capitalise upon.

The existence of interprofessional stereotypes among health- and social-care professionals has been demonstrated in a number of studies. These studies have examined the stereotypes held of other professions by health- and social-care students in relation to interprofessional education. The stereotypes identified by the students are consistent in most of the studies regardless of the stage of training.

These stereotypes included:

- medical students being identified as being low on communication skills (Carpenter, 1995; Barnes *et al.*, 2000; Hean *et al.*, 2006)
- medical students being rated as academically superior (Carpenter, 1995; Barnes *et al.*, 2000; Tunstall-Pedoe *et al.*, 2003; Hean *et al.*, 2006)

- medical students being rated as high on leadership skills (Barnes *et al.*, 2000; Hean *et al.*, 2006)
- nurses, midwives and social workers identified as being high on communication skills (Carpenter, 1995; Tunstall-Pedoe *et al.*, 2003; Hean *et al.*, 2006)
- pharmacists being low on communication skills (Hind *et al.*, 2003; Hean *et al.*, 2006).

The tensions arising from health- and social-care professionals holding these stereotypical beliefs could detract from effective health- and social-care delivery. These stereotypical perceptions that health- and social-care professionals have of each other will impact negatively on both interprofessional teamwork and on the quality of communication. If interprofessional working is to be effective, it is essential that the stereotypical perceptions held by health- and social-care students are challenged.

Evidence base

Find out more about professional stereotyping by reading the following articles.

Mandy, A., Milton, C. and Mandy, P. (2004). Professional Stereotyping and Interprofessional Education. *Learning in Health and Social Care*, **3**(3): 154–170.

Hind, M., Norman, I., Cooper, S., Gill, E., Hilton, R., Judd, P. and Jones, C.J. (2003) Interprofessional Perceptions of Health Care Students. *Journal of Interprofessional Care*, **17**(1): 19–32.

Hean, S., Macleod Clark, J., Adams, K., Humphries, D. and Lathlean, J. (2006) Being Seen by Others as we see Ourselves. The Congruence between in-group and out-group Perceptions of Health and Social Care Students. *Learning in Health and Social Care*, **5**(1): 10–22.

Solutions

Interprofessional education

Since 2004, it has been a requirement that pre-registration health- and social-care programmes across England must provide interprofessional education opportunities for all health- and social-care students. The overarching aim of interprofessional education is to ensure that students learn with, from and about each other to facilitate collaboration in practice (CAIPE, 1997). Expected outcomes and effects of interprofessional education specifically related to professional stereotyping include:

- Self-questioning of personal prejudice and stereotyped views (Parsell *et al.*, 1998)
- Modification of attitudes/perceptions: changes in reciprocal attitudes or perceptions between those groups participating in interprofessional education (Carpenter, 1995; Freeth *et al.*, 2002).

Interprofessional education provides a safe environment in which students can explore and discuss with each other their professional biases and gain an appreciation of professional differences. Part of this exploration will involve the student developing a growing awareness of self.

It is important, however, to remember that professional stereotyping can have positive as well as negative outcomes on interprofessional working. The potential positive outcomes relate to intergroup relations. A number of social science theories have been developed to explain intergroup working and are particularly useful for understanding the complexities of interprofessional working and education.

These theories include:

- **Contact theory**. This theory assumes that contact between members of different groups helps them to discover mutual similarities and positively changes stereotypical attitudes towards each other (Carpenter and Hewstone, 1996).
- **Realistic contact theory**. This theory predicts that where groups hold divergent objectives they will have hostile and discriminatory intergroup relationships, whereas where groups have common objectives, conciliatory behaviour between groups will emerge (Hind *et al.*, 2003).
- **Social identity theory**. This theory is based on the idea that individuals derive their definition of self from their group memberships. Social identity is the identification of self in terms of one's own social group (known as the in-group) rather than of another group (known as the out-group). In the health- and social-care context, this would mean that individual practitioners would define themselves as not only individuals, that is, 'I' or 'me', but also according to the profession to which they belong, that is, 'we social workers', 'we nurses' (Hind *et al.*, 2003).

When members of the different social groups interact, they make comparisons between the characteristics of their own group (the in-group) and the characteristics of the other social group with whom they are interacting (the out-group). In this way, group members establish their identity of self. This comparison is called intergroup differentiation and can be monitored by considering the stereotypes that individuals hold of their own group and those they hold of the out-group (Hean *et al.*, 2006).

So, how can we use the social identity theory and positive stereotyping to help inform interprofessional working and interprofessional education? To ensure positive relations between interacting social groups, for example doctors and nurses, pharmacists and doctors, nurses and radiographers, it is important that when group members are making their intergroup comparisons they are able to see themselves and members of their ingroup as distinctive from other groups (the out-groups) on some characteristics. In a study undertaken by Hean *et al.* (2006), nursing students identified themselves as distinctive on characteristics that included interpersonal skills, team players and practical skills. In the same study, medical students saw their distinctive characteristics as academic ability, leadership, working independently, decision-making and confidence. Social-work students saw themselves as distinct in interpersonal skills, leadership ability and as team players. If group members fail to perceive themselves as distinct, this may lead to an exaggerated favouritism of the in-group and discrimination against the out-group.

Applying this to an interprofessional educational activity, it can be seen that it is important that professional boundaries are maintained. This will ensure that the distinctiveness of each professional group involved in the activity is retained, facilitating harmonious intergroup relations. The outcome of this will be that students should experience good interprofessional relations and will learn that different professions can get on and as a result stereotypical views of each other may become more positive (Carpenter and Hewstone, 1966).

If a group's distinctiveness is threatened, this may result in intergroup conflict. This may occur if there is a disagreement between the stereotypes that students hold of their in-group and the stereotypes held of this group by students of other professions. In Hean *et al.*'s (2006) study, for example, while occupational therapy students believed their group were distinctive on characteristics of interpersonal skills and being team players, this did not match the perceptions of other students. Similarly, radiography students perceived themselves as being distinctive on skills of decision-making and being a team player, but these strengths were not perceived by other students. This would suggest that in the examples given, occupational therapy students and radiography students could potentially experience interprofessional conflict during an interprofessional educational activity.

The ability to identify areas of potential interprofessional conflict is important if interprofessional education is to achieve its overall aim of promoting effective interprofessional working. It is, however, equally important to identify situations where other student groups (out-groups) have more positive perceptions of a particular group than its members (in-group). In these circumstances, unrealistic expectations could be placed on each other during an interprofessional activity. Hean *et al.* (2006) found that other professional groups had positive perceptions of the interpersonal skills of nurses. They suggest that this may lead students from other professions to expect student nurses to be more skilled as communicators and team players than the nurses can demonstrate. This could potentially lead to frustration and anxiety during group activities.

It can be seen that applying the social identity theory to group interactions within an interprofessional context is useful for enhancing our understanding about interprofessional learning processes, the potential positive outcomes of professional stereotyping and the development of effective collaboration in practice.

Lack of willingness to collaborate

To effectively implement collaborative practice, health- and social-care professionals must be willing to commit to a collaborative process. There are a number of reasons why individuals may lack a willingness to collaborate, including lack of agreement on the aims of the team or over-ambitious aims; lack of commitment and support from leaders of the team or organisation; perceived lack of time for collaboration; lack of shared common goals by team members; lack of clearly stated objectives for the team and lack of group cohesion, due to a lack of professional consistency in the team.

Solutions

Effective team building

Team building will facilitate the development of an effective interprofessional team, whereby health- and social-care professionals are willing to engage in collaborative practice. It is important, therefore, that team leaders expend both time and energy in building a team. Team building is not a one-off activity but is a continuous process that not only requires commitment from the team leader but also from all the team members.

Factors that will encourage individuals to participate and make a commitment to interprofessional collaboration include:

- shared common goals which are clear and achievable
- open communication between team members and between team members and the team leader
- a supportive transformational team leader
- time to attend interprofessional education courses/study days/conferences
- time for dialogue and discussion, for example team meetings
- morale support and team spirit
- the roles and responsibilities of team members being clearly articulated and understood by all the team members
- all team members participating fully in the team's activities.

Lack of trust

Trust is one of the key elements required for the development of collaborative practice. Building trust requires time, effort, patience and previous positive experiences. Henneman *et al.* (1995) identify two levels of trust: at one level, trust is about having confidence in your own role and abilities as a professional, while at another level it is about demonstrating trust towards other professionals. At both levels of trust, that trust depends on skills and knowledge, that is, competence and experience of the professional. Within an interprofessional practice environment, professionals place more trust in other professionals considered to be the most experienced and competent.

A lack of trust between members of an interprofessional team will mean that full use of all the knowledge, skills and experience available within the team will not be made. The team will, therefore, not work as effectively as it might and the health and/or social care provided by the team may be compromised as a result.

Lack of trust may also lead to resistance toward the inclusion of team members on patient cases. Each profession may want to handle the case on its own without fully involving the other team members, because of their lack of understanding of what the other professions can offer.

Lack of trust may also result in a team member hesitating to share professional knowledge with the rest of the team. This will alienate and disempower certain team members, which will adversely affect interprofessional working and the delivery of high-quality patient care. Team members' lack of willingness to share professional knowledge may be due, in part, to a desire on the part of the practitioner to defend their own professional identity (see the section on professional tribes on page 135).

Solutions

There are a number of strategies which can be used to facilitate the development of trust between different health- and social-care professions.

Interprofessional learning

Interprofessional learning for health- and social-care practitioners whether at pre-registration or post-registration level, qualificatory or non-qualificatory, in the academic and/or practice setting will enable practitioners to:

- increase their knowledge of the range of skills of others (Parsell *et al.*, 1998)
- understand the roles and responsibilities of other health- and social-care professionals (Parsell *et al.*, 1998; Finch, 2000; Guest *et al.*, 2003)
- gain perspectives of other professionals (Parsell *et al.*, 1998).

Recognition of the expertise of team members

This can be achieved by the team leader establishing an environment in which team members respect one another's knowledge and learn to value one another's differences, so that they are able to build on one another's strengths. In an environment that is supportive of diversity, team members will develop trust in each other and as a result work more effectively together.

Orientation to the role of each profession

When a new member joins an interprofessional team, as part of their induction programme, they should be provided with an insight into the roles and responsibilities of the different professionals within the team. This could be achieved by the new member of staff spending a specified period of time shadowing each different professional within the team. Such a process will increase the level of trust that the new member develops with their team members, which will facilitate collaborative practice.

Reflective activity

Think about when you joined a new team and consider the following points.

- What level of trust did you show towards other professionals within the team?
- What level of trust did the other professionals within the team demonstrate towards you?
- When you joined the team, did lack of trust impact on your ability to work effectively within the interprofessional team?
- How did you develop your knowledge and understanding of the roles and responsibilities of the different professionals within the team?

Lack of communication

Effective communication is an essential precursor for the development of collaboration among health- and social-care professionals. There are three main reasons why communication is considered crucial to effective interprofessional collaboration:

- Professionals must have the ability to communicate to other professionals how their individual and professional competence and experience contribute to the patient outcomes and to the overall achievement of the team's shared goals and objectives.
- Effective communication will enable constructive negotiations with other professionals. When working collaboratively, it is important that professionals are able to explore the situation and find a solution that is acceptable not only to the professionals involved but that is also consistent with the team's philosophy, shared goals and objectives. The best approach for negotiation within a team is to adopt a win-win approach, that is, one in which both parties feel positive about the situation when the negotiation is concluded. This will help to maintain a positive working relationship afterwards.

- Communication – open and active communication and active listening – is crucial for other factors which influence successful collaboration, for example mutual respect, sharing or mutual trust.

Lack of communication between health- and social-care professionals can be due to various reasons. Professionals may perceive that they lack the time required to communicate effectively, for example pressure of the workplace preventing attendance at meetings, or the ability to actively listen to a colleague. Poor negotiation skills may lead to tensions between individual health- and social-care practitioners and may also affect the dynamics of the team. For example, with an overly aggressive approach you may overpower the other person to give you what you want whether or not that is in the patient's or team's best interest. This would clearly be damaging to subsequent teamwork. With a too passive approach, you may simply give in to the other person's wishes. This would clearly not be good for the individual professional.

Information overload, incomplete messages or complex lengthy messages all result in poor communication between different health- and social-care professionals and between health- and social-care professionals and their patients. This has the potential to lead to errors in the care and treatment patients receive (see Chapter 4).

Solutions

Communication skills training for all health- and social-care professionals

Since 2002 all pre-registration health- and social-care students must be able to demonstrate competence in communication with patients, fellow professionals and other health- and social-care staff (Department of Health, 2000). It is important that communication skills training does not stop once the professional has qualified, but continues throughout their professional life.

Interprofessional education

Most universities have adopted an interprofessional learning approach towards the development of communication skills at a pre-registration level. Using a patient-centred approach, students are able to learn from and with each other about the advantages and tensions of interprofessional communication in a safe environment.

The introduction of interprofessional practice placements for pre-registration students also enhances communication with and between health- and social-care professionals, patients and carers.

Students speaking

Behnaz, a second-year adult nursing student, talks about her experiences of completing an interprofessional practice placement within a stroke rehabilitation unit.

This placement provided me with the opportunity to work closely with a number of different professionals, occupational therapists, physios, and speech and language therapists. Before this placement, I knew very little about what an OT or physio did, but now I have a much better understanding and would feel more confident liaising with them in the future.

The MDT meetings were excellent; you learn such a lot listening to the professionals discussing each patient. It makes you realise how important interprofessional communication is, it is essential if the patient is going to receive high-quality care.

This placement has been so valuable to me, it has helped me to consider the 'wider' picture when caring for patients. I will now feel much happier and more confident to liaise and discuss patients' progress with other professionals and recognise the value of their opinions.

ᴿᴿᴿᴿᴿ*Rapid recap*

Check your progress so far by working through each of the following questions.

1. What are the five factors that contribute to effective interprofessional working?
2. What are the three elements that determine how collaboration develops within health- and social-care teams?
3. What type of organisational structure needs to be in place if interprofessional working is to be successful?
4. What team resources need to be available if interprofessional working is to be successful?

If you have difficulty with more than one of the questions, read through the section again to refresh your understanding before moving on.

References

Barnes, D., Carpenter, J. and Dickinson, C. (2000) Interprofessional Education for Community Mental Health: Attitudes to Community Care and Professional Stereotypes. *Social Work Education*, **19**: 565–583.

Blair, T. (1997) Forward. In Secretary of State for Health (1997). *The New NHS: Modern – Dependable*. The Stationery Office, London. Available from: www.dh.gov.uk.

CAIPE (1997) Interprofessional Education – A Definition. *CAIPE Bulletin*, 13.

Carpenter, J. (1995) Doctors and Nurses: Stereotypes and Stereotype Change in Interprofessional Education. *Journal of Interprofessional Care*, **9**(2): 151–161.

Carpenter, J. and Hewstone, M. (1996) Shared Learning for Doctors and Social Workers: Evaluation of a Programme. *The British Journal of Social Work*, **26**(2): 239–257.

Clouder, L. (2003) Becoming Professional: Exploring the Complexities of Professional Socialisation in Health and Social Care. *Learning in Health and Social Care*, **2**(4): 213–222.

D'Amour, D. and Oandasan, I. (2005) Interprofessionality as the Field of Interprofessional Practice and Interprofessional Education: An Emerging Concept. *Journal of Interprofessional Care*, **19**(1): 8–20.

Department of Health (2000) *A Health Service of All the Talents: Developing the NHS Workforce*. HMSO, London. Available from: www.dh.gov.uk.

Dombeck, M. (1997) Professional Personhood: Training, Territoriality and Tolerance. *Journal of Interprofessional Care*, **11**(1): 9–21.

Etzioni, A. (1969) *The Semi-professions and their Organisation*. Free Press, New York.

Finch, J. (2000) IPE and Teamworking – A View from the Education Providers. *BMJ*, **321**: 1138–1140.

Freeth, D., Hammick, M., Koppel, I., Reeves, S. and Barr, H. (2002) *A Critical Review of Evaluations of Interprofessional Education*. Learning and Teaching Support Network (LSTN). Centre for Health Sciences and Practice, Kings College London, London. Available from: www.ltsnhsap.kcl.ac.uk/publications/occasionalpaper/occasionalpaper02.pdf.

General Medical Council. (2001) *Good Medical Practice*. General Medical Council, London. Available from: www.gmc-uk.org.

General Social Care Council (2002) *Code of Practice for Social Care Workers and Employers*. GSCC, London.

Gross, R., McIlveen, R., Coolican, H., Clamp, A. and Russell, J. (2000) *Psychology: A New Introduction for A2*. Hodder and Stoughton, London.

Guest, C., Smith, I., Bradshaw, M. and Hardcastle, W. (2003) Facilitating Interprofessional Learning for Medical and Nursing Students in Clinical Practice. *Learning in Health and Social Care*, **1**: 132–138.

Haslam, S.A., Powell, C. and Turner, J.C. (2000) Social identity, Self-categorisation, and Work Motivation: Rethinking the Contribution of the Group to Positive and Sustainable Organisational Outcomes. *Applied Psychology: An International Review*, **49**: 319–339.

Health Professions Council (2003) *Standards of Conduct, Performance and Ethics*. HPC, London. Available from: www.hpc-uk.org.

Hean, S., Macleod Clark, J., Adams, K., Humphries, D., and Lathlean, J. (2006) Being Seen by Others as we see Ourselves. The Congruence Between in-group and out-group Perceptions of Health and Social Care Students. *Learning in Health and Social Care*, **5**(1): 10–22.

Henneman, E.A., Lee, J.L. and Cohen, J.I. (1995) Collaboration: A Concept Analysis. *Journal of Advanced Nursing*, **23**: 103–109.

Hewison, A. and Sim, J. (1998) Managing Interprofessional Working: Using Codes of Ethics as a Foundation. *Journal of Interprofessional Care*, **12**(3): 309–321.

Hind, M., Norman, I., Cooper, S., Gill, E., Hilton, R., Judd, P. and Jones S.C. (2003) Interprofessional Perceptions of Health Care Students. *Journal of Interprofessional Care*, **17**(1): 19–32.

Kenny, G. (2002a) Children's Nursing and Interprofessional Collaboration: Challenges and Opportunities. *Journal of Clinical Nursing*, **11**(3): 306–312.

Kenny, G. (2002b) 'Interprofessional Working: Opportunities and Challenges. *Nursing Standard*, **17**(6): 33–36.

Lupton, C. and Khan, P. (1998) The Role of Health Professional in the UK Child Protection System: A Literature Review. *Journal of Interprofessional Care*, **12**(2): 209–221.

Mandy, A., Milton, C. and Mandy, P. (2004) Professional Stereotyping and Interprofessional Education. *Learning in Health and Social Care*, **3**(3): 154–170.

Martin-Rodriguez, L.S., Beaulieu, M., D'Amour, D. and Ferrada-Videla, M. (2005) The Determinants of Successful Collaboration: A Review of Theoretical and Empirical Studies. *Journal of Interprofessional Care*, **19**(1): 132–147.

Nursing and Midwifery Council (2002) *Code of Professional Conduct.* NMC, London. Available from: www.nmc-uk.org.

Parsell, G., Spalding, R. and Bligh, J. (1998) Shared Goals, Shared Learning: Evaluation of a Multiprofessional Course for Undergraduate Students. *Medical Education*, **32**(3): 304–311.

Reese, D.J. and Sontag, M. (2001) Successful Interprofessional Collaboration on the Hospice Team. *Health & Social Work*, **26**(3): 167–176.

Reeves, S. and Lewin, S. (2004) Interprofessional Collaboration in the Hospital: Strategies and Meaning. *Journal of Health Services Research & Policy*, **9**(4): 218–226.

Rushmer, R. and Pallis, G. (2002) Interprofessional Working: The Wisdom of Integrated Working and the Disaster of Blurred Boundaries. *Public Money & Management,* October–December, pp. 59–66.

Salvage, J. and Smith, R. (2000) Doctors and Nurses: Doing it Differently. *BMJ*, **320**: 1019–1020.

Secretary of State for Health (1997) *The New NHS, Modern – Dependable.* The Stationery Office, London. Available from: www.dh.gov.uk.

Tunstall-Pedoe, S., Rink, E. and Hilton, S. (2003) Student Attitude to Undergraduate Interprofessional Education. *Journal of Interprofessional Care*, **17**: 161–172.

Woods, B. (2000) *Basics in Psychology.* Hodder and Stoughton, London.

Zelek, B. and Phillips, S.P. (2003) Gender and Power: Nurses and Doctors in Canada. *International Journal for Equity in Health*, 2.

Appendix: Rapid recap answers

Chapter 1

1. **What are the three levels that health- and social-care professionals need to work together at if interprofessional working is to be successful?**

   The three levels at which health- and social-care professionals need to work together if interprofessional working is to be successful are:

   - At a strategic level, agencies are required to plan together and share information about the use of their resources
   - At the level of operational management, a range of policies are required that demonstrate partnership
   - At the level of individual care and support, for example people expect a single point of access into the health care system; shared information systems for interprofessional teams; and joint training.

2. **What is the difference between interprofessional working and multiprofessional working?**

   The difference between interprofessional working and multiprofessional working is that with interprofessional working, professionals work together for the mutual benefit of all the professional groups involved. With multiprofessional working, professionals work or learn side by side for a specific task with little collaboration.

3. **What is interprofessional education?**

   Interprofessional education is when two or more professions learn from and about each other to improve collaboration and the quality of care.

4. **What is interagency working?**

   Interagency working denotes the reciprocal relationship both between and amongst an organisation providing a particular service.

Chapter 2

1. **What are the five drivers for interprofessional working?**

   The drivers for interprofessional working are:

   - The changing health- and social-care environment
   - New government policies and initiatives
   - High-profile child-abuse cases
   - Professional developments
   - Technological developments.

2. **What three factors are still inhibiting successful interprofessional working?**

   The three factors that are inhibiting successful interprofessional working are:

   - Lack of collaboration between agencies
   - Lack of effective communication
   - Lack of adequate training.

3. **What was the purpose of developing Health Action Zones?**

   The purpose of a Health Action Zone was to act as a catalyst to bring together in a working partnership all those contributing to the health of their local population, for example health organisations, local authorities, community groups, voluntary and private sectors, to implement locally agreed strategies for health.

4. **What three main Department of Health policies have impacted on the delivery of stroke services in the UK?**

   The three Department of Health policies that have impacted on the delivery of stroke services in the UK are:

   - *The National Service Framework (NSF) for Older People* (Department of Health, 2001)

- *Saving lives: Our Healthier Nation* (Department of Health, 1999).
- *The National Service Framework for Coronary Heart Disease* (Department of Health, 2001).

Chapter 3

1. What are the essential features of a team?

The essential features of a team are a group of people who:

- Share a common purpose and common goals
- Have a clear understanding of each other's roles and abilities
- Are task oriented and have different but complementary skills
- Have a shared knowledge, skills and resource base and collective responsibility for the outcome of their decisions.

2. What are the essential characteristics of teamwork?

The essential characteristics of teamwork are:

- Having a common purpose and common objectives
- Delegation and empowerment
- Different professional contributions
- Having systems in place to facilitate effective communication
- Coordination, cooperation and joint thinking
- Focusing on the patient to provide the best means of serving the patient's interests
- Allowing team members to carry out the team's work and to manage itself as an independent group of people.

3. What are the five stages of team development?

The five stages of team development are:

- Forming
- Storming
- Norming
- Performing
- Adjourning.

4. List Belbin's nine team roles, which he considered were necessary if a team was to be successful.

Belbin's nine team roles which he considered were necessary if a team was to be successful are:

- Implementer
- Shaper
- Plant
- Resource-investigator
- Monitor evaluator
- Team worker
- Completer-finishers
- Coordinator
- Specialist

5. What factors contribute towards effective interprofessional teamwork?

The factors that contribute towards effective interprofessional teamwork are:

- Clear team goal
- Open communication
- Support for innovation
- High levels of participation
- Clear roles and responsibilities
- Competent team members
- Effective time management
- Values diversity
- High level of commitment
- Joint education and training
- Effective conflict resolution
- Moral support and team spirit.

Chapter 4

1. What are the main types of leadership style?

The main types of leadership style are:

- Participative leadership
- Situational leadership
- Transactional leadership
- Transformational leadership
- Charismatic leadership.

2. What leadership styles are usually adopted by an interprofessional team leader?

The leadership styles that are usually adopted by an interprofessional team leader are transformational leadership and transactional leadership.

3. What skills and qualities does an effective team leader possess?

The skills and qualities that an effective team leader possesses are:

Cluster One: Personal Qualities

a) Self-belief

b) Self-awareness

c) Self-management

d) Drive for improvement

e) Personal integrity.

Cluster Two: Setting Direction

a) Seizing the future

b) Intellectual flexibility

c) Broad scanning

d) Political awareness

e) Drive for results.

Cluster Three: Delivering the Service

a) Leading change through people

b) Holding to account

c) Empowering others

d) Effective and strategic influencing

e) Collaborative working.

4. **What are the strands of professional knowledge?**

   The strands of professional knowledge are:
   - Propositional knowledge
   - Personal knowledge
   - Non-propositional knowledge
   - Social knowledge.

5. **List five of the key characteristics of an expert.**

   The key characteristics of an expert are:
   - Experts are knowledgeable and have a deep level of propositional knowledge and a large volume of non-propositional knowledge
   - Experts are reflective practitioners
   - Experts are highly motivated and internally driven
   - Experts excel mainly in their own domain
   - Experts are faster at performing the skills of their domain
   - Experts are fast at solving problems and make few errors
   - Experts value the participation of relevant others in the decision-making process
   - Experts are patient centred
   - Experts share their expertise to help develop expertise in others.

Chapter 5

1. **What are the main methods of verbal communication?**

   The main methods of verbal communication are spoken language and non-verbal actions. These may be in the form of formal and informal communication and direct (face-to-face) verbal communication strategies. Formal strategies include team meetings, ward rounds and multidisciplinary team meetings. Informal communication strategies are more opportunistic and spontaneous.

2. **What are the benefits of multidisciplinary team meetings?**

   The benefits of multidisciplinary team meetings are:
   - Each different professional contributes independently to the diagnostic treatment or care decisions for a patient case
   - They comprise of professionals working across different sector boundaries
   - They ensure that all professionals involved get an equal opportunity to listen and to talk about the patients within their care
   - They ensure that the patient will receive the most suitable care from diagnosis through treatment to follow-up care and support with the least delay. This will contribute to improved patient outcome.

3. **How do electronic single-patient/health records enhance interprofessional communication?**

   Electronic records enhance interprofessional communication because they are easier to read, less bulky and reduce the need for professionals to re-record information that has already been recorded by another professional. Currently different professions use different documentation systems. This results in a variation in the detail of information that is recorded, potentially leading to less than optimal patient care. By standardising the structure and type of information collected to one central source, any duplication of information/treatment will be avoided and the interprofessional team will be able to work together more effectively.

4. **What factors inhibit interprofessional communication?**

   The factors that inhibit interprofessional communication are:
   - Inappropriate channel of communication selected, for example selecting a written method

when face-to-face communication would have been better or vice versa

- Distractions, for example other people talking, equipment, noise, televisions, radios, interruptions
- Hierarchy – the hierarchical nature of health care creates power gaps that contribute to less than optimal communication between different professionals and with patients
- Lack of time – to communicate effectively takes time and the pressures of the workplace may result in the health care professionals doing another task or thinking about what they are going to do next at the same time as a message is being communicated to them. As a consequence, the health care professional is not fully concentrating and focusing on the person speaking and this may result in vital information being lost or misinterpreted
- Complex messages – these will increase the chances of the message being misunderstood or misinterpreted
- Ideological differences between health care professions
- Too much information – this may result in information overload
- Different professional language
- Different professional jargon
- Too much communication – may be via the telephone or e-mail or during a ward round or team meeting, with so many communications it can be difficult if not impossible to determine which communications are most critical.

Chapter 6

1. What are the key features of a community of practice?

The key features of a community of practice are:

- Communities of practice are everywhere – at home, at work, at university – we all belong to a number of them
- Communities of practice are informally bound by what they do together and by what they have learned through their mutual engagement in these activities
- They develop around things that matter to people

- The practices of a community reflect the members' own understanding of what is important
- Communities of practice are defined by what the community is about; how it functions and what capability it has produced.

2. List the key points of situated learning theory.

The key points of situated learning theory are:

- Situated learning recognises that knowledge is embedded within the context in which it is used and cannot be separated from the activity, context and culture of that situation
- Learners engage in situated learning by negotiating meaning with one another through the use of tools and artefacts such as language, books, music and art
- Learning takes place as a result of participating in 'real' activities that nurture and guide the learner's ability to think
- Learners develop a shared understanding about the purpose of the community and develop a sense of belonging.

3. What are the key features of a situated-learning environment?

The key features of a situated-learning environment are:

- It fosters the development of lifelong learning skills
- Situated learning and teaching strategies include critical appreciation; cooperative learning; collaboration; reflection; coaching and narrative
- Learning takes place in the zone of proximal development through interactions between a newcomer and an old-timer
- Learner and facilitator are actively involved in and jointly manage the responsibility for learning
- Situated learning techniques take more time and effort for both the learner and facilitator.

4. What is the role of an interprofessional mentor?

The primary role of an interprofessional mentor would be the same as those of a uniprofessional mentor, that is, the facilitation of learning, supervision and assessment of learners in the practice environment. The application of these roles, however, would be related to the learner's interprofessional learning outcomes.

Chapter 7

1. **What are the five factors that contribute to effective interprofessional working?**

   The five factors that contribute to effective interprofessional working are:

   - UK health- and social-care policies and legislation
   - Teams, teamwork and team dynamics
   - Leadership and expertise
   - Communicating with each other
   - Interprofessional learning.

2. **What are the three elements that determine how collaboration develops within health- and social-care teams?**

   The three elements which determine how collaboration develops within health- and social-care teams are:

   - Systemic factors – conditions outside the organisation
   - Organisational factors – conditions within organisation

   - Interactional factors – interpersonal relationships between team members.

3. **What type of organisational structure needs to be in place if interprofessional working is to be successful?**

   The type of organisational structure that needs to be in place if interprofessional working is to be successful is a horizontal structure. A horizontal structure, rather than the traditional hierarchical structure, needs to be in place if there is to be successful integrated collaboration between health- and social-care professionals.

4. **What team resources need to be available if interprofessional working is to be successful?**

   The team resources that need to be available if interprofessional working is to be successful are:

   - Regular team meetings to provide an opportunity for the team leaders and team members to meet and communicate face to face about matters that affect the team
   - Allocation of dedicated space.

Index

Page references in *italics* indicate figures or tables

abuse of children 22–4
Access to Health Records Act 1990 99
agency-based working 7
Agenda for Change, Modernising the NHS Pay System (Department of Health, 1999b) 18
agendas, team meeting 89–91
Alma Ata Declaration (World Health Organization, 1978) 14, 46
annual reviews, staff 20

barriers to interprofessional working 131–2
  interactional factors 143–51
  organisational factors 140–3
  systemic factors 132–40
Bass and Avolio's (1994) transformational leadership 61
Belbin's (1981) team roles 39–41, *40*
Benne and Skeats' (1948) team roles 38–9, *38, 39*
Beveridge Report 1942 13
boundaries
between nursing and medical professions 139–40
  establishing clear 136, 147
Bradford, Heath Action Zone 26

Care Trusts 19
Caring for People: Community Care in the Next Decade and Beyond (Department of Health, 1989b) 15
chairperson, role of 91–2, 92–3
charismatic leadership 63–5
child abuse 22–4

Climbié, Victoria 22
  report into death of 23, 82, 108
coaching 118
codes of conduct 137–9
cognitive continuum theory 74–5
collaboration 9, 118
  barriers to 143–51
Colwell, Maria, report into death of 23
Combined Universities Interprofessional Learning Unit (CUILU), interprofessional capability framework, 2004 128
commitment, within teams 52
communication 81
  barriers to 101–3, 134, 142, 151
  and effective teamwork 51
  enabling technologies 97–101
  importance of 150–1
  methods of 83–7
  multidisciplinary team meetings 93–6
  process *102*
  recommendations relating to 81–3
  skills training 151
  team meetings 87–93
  ward rounds 96–7
'communication books' 4
communities of practice 112, 113–15
  frameworks for learning 115–18
  support for learners 122–5
  tools for learning 118–21
community care 15
Computer Misuse Act 1990 99
concept-based working 7
conflict, intergroup 147

conflict resolution, and teamwork 53
Conger and Kanungo's (1998) charismatic leadership 64–5
Connect - the Communication Disability Network 30
contact theory 146
cooperation 9
cooperative learning 116–17
critical appreciation 115–16

Data Protection Act 1998 99
decision making, during meetings 91–2
demographic changes, and health- and social-care 21
Department of Health
  Agenda for Change, Modernising the NHS Pay System, 1999b 18
  Caring for People: Community Care in the Next Decade and Beyond, 1989b 15
  A First Class Service: Quality in the New NHS, 1998b 27
  Health Act - Modern Partnerships for People 1999 17–18
  A Health Service of all the Talents: Developing the NHS Workforce, 2000c 109
  Health- and Social-Care Act 2001 19
  Knowledge and Skills Framework (KSF), 2003 19–20
  Making a Difference: Strengthening the Nursing, Midwifery and Health Visiting Contribution to Health and Health Care, 1999 107, 109

Meeting the Challenge: A Strategy for the Allied Health Professions, 2000b 109, 122
Modernising Social Services, 1998a 16
The NHS Improvement Plan: Putting People at the Heart of Public Services, 2004b 20
NHS Leadership Qualities Framework, 2002 66–7
The NHS Plan: a Plan for Investment, a Plan for Reform, 2000a 19, 81, 109
Saving Lives: Our Healthier Nation, 1999d 30
Working for Patients, 1989a 14
Working Together, Learning Together: A Framework for Lifelong Learning in the NHS, 2001 110
diabetes 2–3
Different Strokes (association) 30
doctor-nurse relationship 140
Dreyfus and Dreyfus (1986) model of skill acquisition 73–4

education
  and effective teamwork 52
  interprofessional *see* interprofessional education
  multiprofessional 11
  EHR (electronic health records) 98
  EPR (electronic patient records) 98
experience
  acquiring knowledge through 70
  and expertise 71, 73
experts and expertise 68
experience and expertise 71–2
  knowledge expertise 75–7
  models for developing expertise 72–5
  professional knowledge 69–71, 69
  recognition of team members' expertise 149

First Class Service, A: Quality in the New NHS (Department of Health, 1998b) 27
formal communication 84
Freedom of Information Act 2000 99

general practitioners, and social services in 1960s 13–14
General Social Care Council (GSCC), code of conduct 138
goals, and effective teamwork 51
government policies and initiatives 13–20, 21–2, 23
grouping 7, 8

Hammond's (1980) cognitive continuum theory 74–5
Health Act 1999 17–18
Health Action Zones (HAZs) 25, 26–7
  Bradford 26
  Luton 25–6
Health Professions Council (HPC), code of conduct 137, 138
Health Service of all the Talents, A: Developing the NHS Workforce (Department of Health 2000c) 109
health services 24
  see also NHS
Health- and Social-Care Act 2001 19
Healthspace website 98–9
Hersey and Blanchard (1977) leadership styles 58–9, 58, 59
high-performance teams 43

identity, professional 136
'illness scripts' 76
informal communication 84
innovation, effective teamwork and 51
integrated care 15, 19
interdependence 141
internal market 14, 15
interprofessional
  defining 6, 9–10
  different from multiprofessional 11
interprofessional capability framework (CUILU, 2004) 128
interprofessional collaboration 10, 118
  barriers to 143–51
interprofessional education
  breaking down barriers 134, 145–7, 149, 151
  definition of 10
  drivers for 107–10

frameworks for 115–18
  situated learning 111–15
  support for learners 122–8
  and teamwork 52
  tools for 118–21
interprofessional mentorship 126–8
interprofessional teamwork *see* teams and teamwork
interprofessional working
  barriers to 23, 131–51
  development of 13–20
  drivers of 21–5
  initiatives encouraging 25–30
  three levels of 1
intuition 74

jargon 103

Katzenbach and Smith's (1993) model of team types 42–3, 43
knowledge
  and expertise 75–7
  professional 69–71, 69
Knowledge and Skills Framework (KSF), NHS 19–20

Labonte, Ainlee, report into death of 23
language, differences in professional 11, 134
Lave and Wenger's (1991) theory of situated learning 111–15
leadership
  definitions of 55
  effective team leaders 65–7
  ineffective leaders 141
  styles 56–65
  trait theory of 56, 56
learning *see* interprofessional education
learning outcomes 127–8
'legitimate peripheral participation' 111, 112, 113
Luton, Health Action Zone 25–6

Making a Difference: Strengthening the Nursing, Midwifery and Health Visiting Contribution to Health and Health Care (Department of Health, 1999) 107, 109
managers, first-level 60
Margerison and McCann's (1995) team roles 41, 41

MDTs *see* multidisciplinary teams
medical profession, and nursing profession 139–40
Meeting the Challenge: A Strategy for the Allied Health Professions (Department of Health, 2000b) 109, 122
meetings
 and differing schedules 143
 and effective teamwork 52
 multidisciplinary teams 93–6
 regular 142
 team 87–93
 ward rounds 96–7
mentors and mentoring 122–3
 definition of mentoring 123–4
 history of mentoring 123
 interprofessional mentorship 127–8
 role and characteristics of mentors 124–5, *125*
minutes of meetings 92, 93
mobile carts 97
Modernising Government (National Audit Office, 1999) 17
Modernising Social Services (Department of Health, 1998a) 16
moral support within teams 53
multidisciplinary teams (MDTs) 29, 93–4, *93*, *94*
 meetings 93, 94–6
 use of PACS 100–1
multiprofessional, meaning of term 10–11

narratives 120–1
National Audit Office, *Modernising Government*, 1999 17
National Service Frameworks (NSFs) 17
NSF for Older People 27–8
New NHS, The, Modern - Dependable (Secretary of State for Health, 1997) 15–16
NHS
 formation of 13
 internal market and 14
 Knowledge and Skills Framework 19–20
 modernisation 15–16, 17–18, 19
 modernising pay system 18
 structure of 140–1

NHS and Community Care Act 1990 15
NHS Headings Project (NHS Information Authority, 2003) 99
NHS Improvement Plan, The: Putting People at the Heart of Public Services (Department of Health, 2004b) 20
NHS Leadership Qualities Framework (Department of Health, 2002) 66–7
NHS Plan, The: a Plan for Investment, a Plan for Reform (Department of Health, 2000a) 19, 81, 109
non-verbal communication 83
NSFs (National Service Frameworks) 17
NSF for Older People 27–8
Nursing and Midwifery Council (NMC)
 code of conduct 138
 and mentoring 122, 124, 125
nursing profession, and the medical profession 139–40

O'Neill, Dennis 22
 report into death of 22
organisations 140
 communication within 142
 leadership within 141
 philosophy 141
 schedule and routine differences 143
 structures 140–1
 team resources 141–2
Øvretviet's (1997) model for describing teams 44–5

PACS (picture archiving and communication systems) 100–1
palliative care 49
palliative-care teams 49, *50*
participative leadership 57, *57*
patients
 empowerment 21
 primary health care teams and 48
 records 86–7, 98–100
pay system, new NHS 18
personal development plans 20
personal knowledge 70, 118

philosophy
 diversity of within teams 52, 133–4, *133*
 organisational 141
picture archiving and communication systems (PACS) 100–1
potential teams 43
practical knowledge 69
primary health care teams 46–7, *47*, *48*
problem association 7, 7–8
problem solving, experts and novices 75, 76
process-based working 7
professional, meaning of term 8, 10
professional identity 136
professional knowledge 69–71, *69*
professional system 132
 codes of conduct 137–9
 language 11, 134–5
professional developments 24
professions and professionalisation 8, 10, 139
 socialisation 132–4
 tribes and territories 135–6
propositional and non-propositional knowledge 69–70, *69*
pseudo-teams 42–3

real teams 43
realistic contact theory 146
records, patient 86–7, 98–100
reflection 114, 118–20
resources
 for multidisciplinary team meetings 95–6
 for teams 141–2

Saving Lives: Our Healthier Nation (Department of Health, 1999d) 30
schema theory of expertise 75–7
Schmidt *et al.*'s (1990) four-stage model of medical expertise 76
Secretary of State for Health
 The New NHS, Modern - Dependable, 1997 15–16
 Report into the Death of Victoria Climbié, 2003 23, 82, 108

Report into the Deaths of
  Children from Heart Surgery
  at Bristol Royal Infirmary,
  2001 82, 108
Seebohm Report, 1968 13–14
situated learning 111–12
  criticisms of theory of 113–15
  frameworks for 115–18
  tools for 118–21
situational leadership 57–9
smoking 2
social identity theory 146
social knowledge 70, 118
social services 24
  community care 15
  and GPs in 1960s 13–14
  modernisation 16, 18
social system and interprofessional
    working 139–40
socialisation, professional 132–4
Speakability (charity) 30
specialisation 24
staff meetings *see* team meetings
staff, NHS
  annual reviews 20
  extension of roles 19
  new pay system 18
stereotypes and stereotyping
    144–8
stroke 27
  initiative encouraging
    interprofessional working
    27–30
Stroke Association, The 30

teams and teamwork 9
  defining a team 33–4
  defining teamwork 34
  development of a team 34–6
  diversity of values, philosophies
    and theories within 52, 133–4,
    133
  factors contributing to effective
    51–3, 148
  lack of resources 141–2
  leaders 65–7, 141
  and leadership styles 57, 57–9,
    62, *63*, 64, 65
  meetings 87–93
  models for types of teams 42–5
  multidisciplinary teams 29,
    93–6, *93*, *94*, 100–1
  and NHS Knowledge and Skills
    Framework 20
  palliative-care teams 49, *50*
  primary health care teams 46–7,
    47, *48*
  recognition of expertise of
    members 149
  roles within teams 37–41, *38*,
    39, *40*, *41*, 51–2, 150
technical knowledge 69
technology 97–8
  developments in 25
  electronic records 98–100
  picture archiving and
    communication systems 100–1
  and ward rounds 97
territories 135

trait theory of leadership 56, *56*
transactional leadership 60, 62–3,
    63
transformational leadership 61–2,
    62–3, *63*
tribes 135
trust 148–9
  development of 149–50
  lack of 149

values, diversity of within teams
    52, 133, *133*
verbal communication 83–5
videoconferencing 95, 143

ward rounds 96–7
workforce, NHS
  annual reviews 20
  extension of roles 19
  new pay system 18
working groups 42
Working for Patients (Department
    of Health, 1989a) 14
*Working Together, Learning
    Together: A Framework for
    Lifelong Learning in the NHS*
    (Department of Health, 2001)
    110
World Health Organization, Alma
    Ata Declaration, 1978 14, 46
written communication 85–6
  patient records 86–7, 98–100

zone of proximal development 70